W9-DCM-586

Basic Cardiology

A guide to important principles

Basic
Cardiology

David Verel
MD FRCP
*Consultant Cardiologist to the Sheffield
Regional Hospital Board and United
Sheffield Hospitals
Lecturer in Cardiology
University of Sheffield*

A Chapter on
Surgical Intensive Care

G. H. Smith
MB FRCS
*Consultant Cardio-thoracic Surgeon
to the Sheffield Regional Hospital Board
and United Sheffield Hospitals,
Lecturer in Cardio-thoracic Surgery
University of Sheffield*

ḦḦ

Published, in association with
Hastings Hilton Publishers Limited,
by

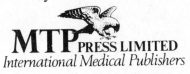

MTP **PRESS LIMITED**
International Medical Publishers

Published, in association with
Hastings Hilton Publishers Limited
London,
by

MTP Press Limited
International Medical Publishers
Head Office:
Falcon House, Lancaster
England LA1 1PE

This edition published in 1979

Copyright © MCMLXXIII David Vérel,
under the original title of *Essential
Cardiology*

ISBN 0 85200 047 2

*No part of this book may be reproduced
in any form without permission from the
publishers except for the quotation of
brief passages for the purposes for review*

Printed in Great Britain

Contents

Preface

The very rapid advances in technology have caused a revolution in Nursing practice in the last ten years. We are now only twelve years from the first description of permanent cardiac pacing. This is now an accepted method of treatment throughout the world. Bedside monitoring with oscilloscopes has passed from being an experimental investigation to normal ward practice. This rapid invasion has involved technicians and nursing staff in matters which until comparatively recently were regarded as the province of the Specialist Doctor. This book is intended primarily to give an introduction to the subject to nurses and technicians concerned with Intensive Care techniques. It is hoped it may also be of interest to Medical Students as an introduction to the subject and also as a review to those preparing for examinations.

Sheffield, September 1972.   David Vérel

Introduction

About one third of deaths today are due to disease of the heart and circulation. This alone would justify a special study of them by nurses and doctors. They are of particular importance to nurses, however, as there is no other group of diseases where quick informed action by a nurse in an emergency, can save so many lives. In this book the functions of the heart and circulation are first described. There follows a brief account of the diseases of the heart, and finally, intensive coronary care and intensive post-operative care are dealt with in some detail. For this it is necessary to have some familiarity with monitoring and resuscitive equipment. The workings of this type of equipment are therefore described at the end of the book.

FUNCTION OF THE HEART

The heart is a double pump which pumps blood round the body, back to the heart and then pumps it again through the lungs. In an average man each side of the heart pumps out about 5 litres of blood each minute. If the heart rate is 70 beats per minute, the heart will pump out 5,000 ÷ 70 ml blood per beat, or about 70 ml at each beat. This is about a tea cupful at each beat to the lungs and to the body.

The circulation

The circulation of the blood to all parts of the body is like the traffic in a small town. In a town all sorts of things are going on simultaneously, with certain types of activity predominating at different times. We may think of some of these for a moment, for the complex happenings in a town are very like those that depend on the circulation. In the morning of a working day, buses and cars will be taking people to different places connected with their work, to go shopping or to see friends. Other vehicles will be delivering goods to shops, others collecting refuse. The electricity and gas works will be generating power from fuel brought by ship or train. Policemen will be directing traffic, courts dealing with malefactors and doctors and nurses helping the sick. It is possible to get a clear picture of what is happening at one place at one time, but the whole story is too big and too complicated to be seen all at once.

We have the same difficulty with the body and its circulation. The circulation is shown diagrammatically in Fig.1. If we start with the aorta, blood from this is distributed to the limbs, the brain, the gut, kidneys, liver, and spleen. Some of this blood returns directly to the heart, but most of the blood which has passed through the gut and spleen, is passed through the liver before returning to the heart.

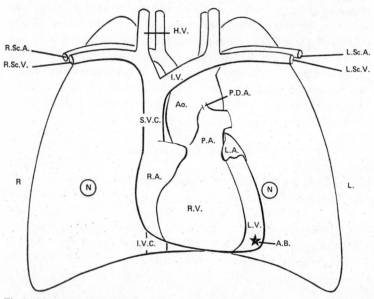

Fig.1. Diagram of the heart seen from the front with the chest open. HV neck vessels, RScA right subclavian artery, RScV right subclavian vein, LScA left subclavian artery, LScV left subclavian vein, IV innominate vein, SVC superior vena cava, AO aorta, PA pulmonary artery, PDA patent ductus arteriosus, RA right atrium, LA left atrium, N nipple, RV right ventricle, LV left ventricle, IVA inferior vena cava, AB apex beat, R right, L left.

Note that the heart is viewed as though seen by someone looking from the front, the right side being on the left, and the left side being on the right.

Here it collects in the right atrium, passes to the right ventricle, which pumps the blood to the pulmonary artery. It then passes through the capillaries of the lungs and collects in the left atrium before entering the left ventricle to be pumped to the aorta. Note that blood is supplied to the heart itself by two arteries which leave the aorta at its beginning. These are the coronary arteries (so called because they resemble a royal crown). Some of this blood returns to the right atrium by the coronary sinus (the vein of the heart) and some re-enters the heart directly by veins in the muscles of the ventricles.

We may now return to our analogy with the traffic in a town. The blood consists of a very complex kind of traffic which includes fuel, oxygen, waste products, building materials, finished and half finished products, repair gangs, demolition men and messenger boys, all visiting sooner or later every part of the town. The main activity depends upon the place the blood is passing through. In the kidney the blood is filtered, in the liver the digestive products are dealt with, either being stored or treated chemically before being passed on to their ultimate destination. In the spleen, among other things, worn out red cells are collected and scrapped, and antibodies manufactured. In the lungs, oxygen and carbon dioxide are exchanged. Just as the traffic pattern in a town changes, for example in a rush hour, so does the pattern of the circulation. While walking, more blood is passed through the leg arteries to supply fuel and remove waste products there. After meals the gut arteries open up and more blood flows through the abdomen to cope with digestion. At night the heart slows down in sleep and the output is cut to a minimum. No man-made pump can approach its reliability.

1

Anatomy of the heart

EMBRYOLOGY

The heart starts as a single tube. In the course of the first three months of intra-uterine life, it develops into the two atria and ventricles, connected to the appropriate veins and arteries. The partitions (septa) which divide the original tube into the two separate sides of the heart, grow simultaneously in different parts of the tissue which is to become the heart. It is therefore not surprising that these septa do not always meet successfully, and so holes (defects) are left. Similarly the development of the valves may be faulty and the connections between the arteries and veins may be incorrect.

Compared with most other animals, man's chest is wide from side to side and very shallow from front to back. In most animals, such as the cat or dog, the heart lies much more in the centre than is possible in man; the ventricles, in particular, being nearly on the right and left of the mid-line. This is not possible in man, and the ventricles have to grow over to one side in order to fit in. Usually the ventricles grow over to the left (*laevocardia*), with the result that the right ventricle comes to lie much more in front of the left ventricle, than to the right side, and the left ventricle lies much more to the back (posterior) of the right ventricle, than it does to the left. We may, therefore, speak of the anterior ventricle instead of the right, or the posterior ventricle instead of the left. In some congenital heart conditions in which the ventricles have developed in the wrong way, it may be less ambiguous to speak of them in this way.

On rare occasions, a normal heart, instead of going to the left, goes to the right (*dextrocardia*). In such people, who are usually otherwise quite normal, the abdominal contents are also often on the wrong sides, the liver on the left, stomach on the right and appendix on the left. This is called *situs inversus*.

The heart may develop abnormally with its main bulk on the right, but the two atria in their correct positions. This may be called *dextrocardia* but is usually termed dextro-position.

ANATOMY OF THE HEART AND GREAT VESSELS

The plan the heart works on is simple enough. On both sides blood flows from the veins into the collecting chambers called the atria, then passes through non-return valves into the high pressure chambers called the ventricles. These contract and force the blood through non-return valves into the great arteries to the body and lungs. It is, however, surprisingly difficult to get a clear picture in the mind of how the various parts lie relative to one another. As the relations of the various parts are important in understanding heart disease, they will be briefly described. (The word 'relations' is used in a technical sense in medical writing, to mean the structures adjacent to one another. Thus the tip of the tongue is related to the roof of the mouth above, the teeth in front, the floor of the mouth and salivary ducts below, and the rest of the tongue behind when the mouth is closed.)

General appearance

We may begin by describing the general appearance of the intact heart in the thorax (chest). Viewed from the front it resembles a triangle, with the base on the right border of the sternum and the apex at the point on the left, where the apex beat can be felt (Fig.1). These two areas are commonly called the base and the apex respectively. The heart lies in the mediastinum, with the lungs on either side and the diaphragm below. In an x-ray, the shadow of the pulmonary artery (artery to the lungs) can be seen on the left just above the heart, and the aorta (artery to the body) just above the pulmonary artery, also on the left. The apex beat corresponds well with the extent to which the heart extends to the left, and its displacement in heart enlargement is a good measure of the size of the heart.

In considering the plan of the heart we shall take the chambers in pairs, beginning with the atria. In doing so, it will be remembered that the names 'left' and 'right' refer to the development of the heart rather than to their actual positions in the adult.

The atria

The left atrium lies at the back of the heart in a central position (Fig.2). Four large veins enter it, two on each side, bringing arterial blood from the upper and lower parts of each lung respectively. These are called the main pulmonary veins. Immediately behind the centre of the atrium is the oesophagus and behind that the thoracic spine. A finger like extension of the atrium passes forward on the left as a blind sac, called the atrial appendix or auricle. (To add to the confusion over names, people sometimes refer to the whole atrium as the auricle.) Blood leaves the atrium by an opening lying to the left and below, and passes through the mitral valve into the left ventricle. The right atrium lies to the right of the left atrium and somewhat in front of it (Fig.1,2). Blood from the upper part of the body above the diaphragm enters it by a vein called the superior vena cava, and blood from below the diaphragm by the inferior vena cava, which passes behind the diaphragm to enter the right

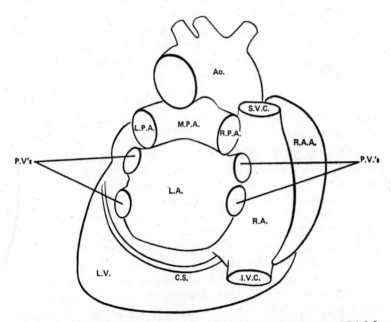

Fig.2. The heart seen from behind removed from the chest. AO aorta, LPA left pulmonary artery, MPA main pulmonary artery, RPA right pulmonary artery, SVC superior vena cava, PVS pulmonary veins, LA left atrium, RA right atrium, RAA right atrial appendix, LV left ventricle, CS coronary sinus, IVC inferior vena cava.

atrium. This atrium also has an auricle which projects forward on the right. The right atrium empties into the right ventricle by way of the tricuspid valve, which lies almost directly on the left at the lower extremity of the atrium. The main vein draining the heart is called the coronary sinus. It enters the atrium just behind the lower extremity of the tricuspid valve.

The two atria are separated by a thin membrane called the atrial septum, in which there is a flap valve which allows blood to go from right to left, but not from left to right. This valve, which is called the foramen ovale or ostium secundum is open in the unborn child when the blood normally passes through it, but is held closed in extra-uterine life by the higher pressure in the left atrium. It is easily opened in most babies, but, by the time a child is a few years old, is usually sealed by fibrous adhesions.

The ventricles

From the atria the blood passes through to the ventricles. These have thick muscular walls, the left ventricular wall being thicker than the right, as might be expected, as it pumps blood at about four times the pressure generated in the right. The valves at the entrance of the ventricles are designed to let the blood flow in easily and then to prevent its return to the atrium.

THE LEFT VENTRICLE. The *mitral valve* of the left ventricle, owes its name to a supposed resemblance to the ceremonial hat of a bishop, the mitre. It is much more like the sort of paper crown that is found in a Christmas cracker. Such a crown could be made by taking a large paper bag, putting it on your head, and then getting a friend to cut the bottom of the bag into large V shaped points. The mitral valve is like such a bag attached all round the opening into the ventricle (Fig.3). The points of the hat end in fine string like cords (called the chordae tendinae), which are attached to the tips of small muscular projections (the papillary muscles) at the apex of the ventricle. The two sides of the valve are pushed aside by the blood entering the ventricle. The blood then flows into the cavity through the gaps beyond the continuous sheet of the valve cusps, and between the cords. When the ventricle contracts the sides of the valve are forced together and the blood cannot get back into the atrium. As the ventricle contracts, it gets shorter, tending to blow the valve inside-out, so that it might be expected to leak. This is prevented by the

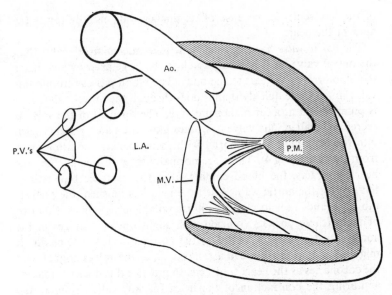

Fig.3. The heart viewed from behind and to the left with the left ventricle opened. PVS pulmonary veins, LA left atrium, MV mitral valve, AO aorta, PM papillary muscles.

The cut surface of the ventricle is shown hatched.

papillary muscles which contract, so pulling on the chordae and keeping the valve from leaking (Fig.3). We shall see that if the chordae break or the papillary muscles are damaged by heart disease, the valve may leak. A valve which is not leaking is called *competent*, while one which is leaking is called *incompetent*. Mitral valve leaking is called *mitral incompetence*. The mitral valve is arranged, like a paper bag, with two sides. These sides are usually called cusps and the valve is said to be bicuspid. One side of the valve is attached along the ventricular septum (the anterior cusp), while the posterior cusp is attached along the outer heart wall. At the upper end, part of the valve attachment shares a bridge of tissue with the aortic valve. This, with the mitral valve, closes the ventricle (Fig.3). The ventricle is therefore like a balloon with the two valves stopping up its entrance, one allowing blood in, the other out. Blood flows into the ventricle from the atrium at the back, fills the ventricle, and then flows back again, through the aortic valve which lies in front of and above the atrium. The ventricle lies at the back of the heart, running forwards, downwards, and to the left. The tip of the left ventricle, because of its thicker wall, usually forms the apex of the heart.

The *aortic valve* has three cusps. It is a much simpler valve than the mitral valve, as it has only to close the large artery which takes the blood from the heart to the body. The blood passes through this valve much more quickly than it does through the mitral valve, as it is pumped out at a far higher pressure. The opening of the valve is therefore smaller. The valve cusps are like little patch pockets sewn into the beginning of the aorta, with their openings pointing away from the heart (Fig.4). There are normally three of them. When the heart contracts, the blood coming from the ventricle blows them flat against the aortic wall. When the beat has finished, the pockets flip open and meet to close the aorta completely. From inside two of them (these pockets coincide with slight outward bulges in the aorta called sinuses of Valsalva) the coronary arteries come off. It might seem that this is a bad arrangement, as the valves might block the coronaries as the heart contracts. In practice this does not matter, as during the contraction of the heart (usually called *systole*), the

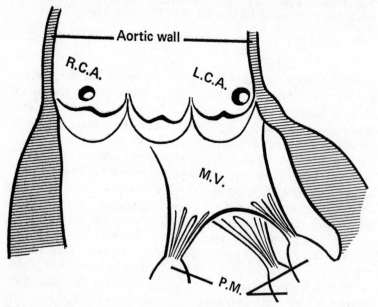

Fig.4. Diagram of the aortic and mitral valves. The aorta has been cut down between the junction of the anterior and the left aortic valve cusps. RCA right coronary artery, LCA left coronary artery, MV mitral valve, PM papillary muscle. The cut surface of the aortic wall and left ventricle is shown hatched.

muscles squeeze so tightly that blood cannot get into the muscle and no coronary flow occurs. When the heart relaxes to fill again (this is called *diastole*), the aortic valves flip shut and the coronary arteries are filled by blood freshly oxygenated by its passage through the lungs.

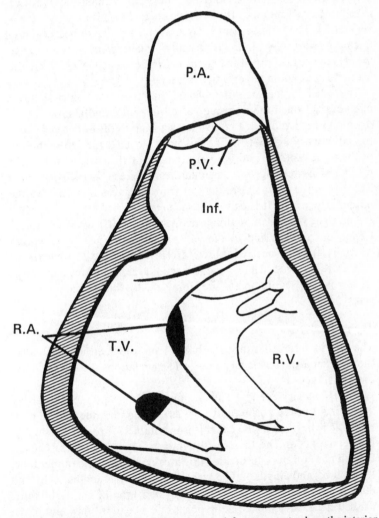

Fig.5. The heart seen from in front and to the left, cut open to show the interior of the right ventricle. PA pulmonary artery, PV pulmonary valve, INF infundib-ulum, TV tricuspid valve, RA right atrium seen through the tricuspid valve, RV right ventricle.

THE RIGHT VENTRICLE. The arrangement for the right ventricle is broadly similar to that of the left with two important differences. The inlet valve to the ventricle has three cusps, not two. It is called the *tricuspid valve*. The cusps end in chordae tendinae and papillary muscles just like those of the left ventricle, but it is easy to see that a valve with three parts would leak more easily than one with two if the pressure went up or the ventricle enlarged. This in fact happens very easily. This enlargement is often temporary due to heart failure. Such temporary leaking is usually called *functional tricuspid incompetence*, in contrast to *organic tricuspid incompetence*, where the leaking is due to damage to the valve.

The other important difference, is that the right ventricle has a main cavity which the tricuspid valve leads into, and a sort of neck or spout like that of a tea pot, which leads up to the outlet valve into the pulmonary artery (Fig.5). This neck is called the infundibulum of the right ventricle and is a very important structure as it is often the site of narrowings in congenital heart disease. A tricuspid valve like that in the aorta closes the exit from the infundibulum into the pulmonary artery. It is called the *pulmonary valve*.

The right ventricle lies along the front of the left ventricle, going, like it, downwards and to the left, separated from it by a septum which is a thick sheet of muscle except just at the top where the valves are attached. Here there is a small area of fibrous membrane which is the commonest site for defects (holes) between the ventricles.

The great arteries

The great arteries that take the blood from the ventricles are called the *aorta* and the *pulmonary artery*. Their relations are important in cardiac surgery.

The pulmonary artery. The beginning of the pulmonary artery lies in front of the aorta and to the left of the mid line (as the right ventricle is in front of the left this is inevitable). It passes backwards for about 3–5 cm and then divides into two main branches. The left branch goes on back to divide into three main branches (upper lobe, lower lobe and lingula). The right branch passes to the right and divides into three branches—one for each lobe of the right lung. These further divide like the branches of a tree, until they end in the alveolar capillaries where the exchange of gases takes place. These in turn drain into a series of veins, getting larger as they join together and end as the four pulmonary veins we began with.

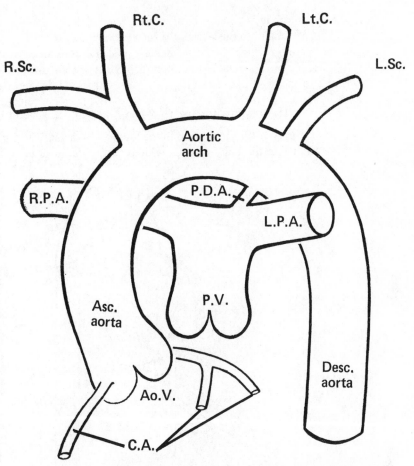

Fig.6. Diagram of the great vessels RtC right carotid artery, LtC left carotid artery, RSc right subclavian artery, LSc left subclavian artery, RPA right pulmonary artery, PDA patent ductus arteriosus, LPA left pulmonary artery, Asc aorta ascending aorta, AoV aortic valve, PV pulmonary valve, Desc aorta descending aorta, CA coronary arteries.

The aorta. The aorta starts on the right of the pulmonary artery and just behind it. It passes forwards (remember the pulmonary artery passed backwards), and to the right. It then loops up in front of the right pulmonary artery, over it, now going to the left and down behind the point where the pulmonary artery divides (bifurcates). At this point, the front of the aorta and the back of the pulmonary artery are joined together by an artery called the *ductus arteriosus*, which is needed while the child is a foetus in the uterus, but which normally closes at birth. We shall be considering the foetal circulation shortly. This remarkable loop which the aorta makes round the pulmonary artery, is called the aortic arch. The main branches of the arch go to the arms and to the head and neck (Fig.6).

THE FOETAL CIRCULATION

The essential features of the circulation in the foetus, are the adjustments made to enable the baby to exist without using its lungs to

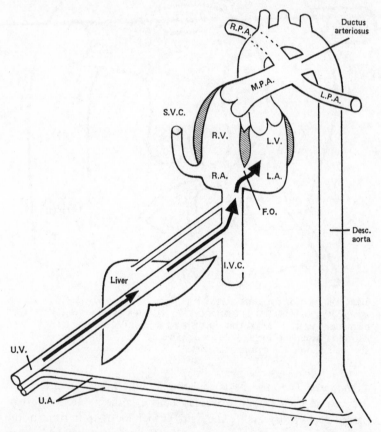

Fig.7. A diagram of the foetal circulation. The main path of blood coming from the mother is shown by the arrows. RPA right pulmonary artery, MPA main pulmonary artery, LPA left pulmonary artery, SVC superior vena cava, RV right ventricle, LV left ventricle, RA right atrium, LA left atrium, FO foramen ovale, IVC inferior vena cava, UV umbilical vein, UA umbilical arteries.

breathe, or its mouth to eat. The placenta which connects the baby to its mother has to perform both these functions, as well as permitting an exchange of waste products, such as carbon dioxide and urea, with the mother's blood. The arrangement is shown, diagrammatically in Fig.7. Oxygenated blood carrying nutrients from the mother comes from the placenta along the umbilical vein, enters the umbilicus, passes to the hepatic vein and enters the inferior vena cava. In the right atrium the foramen ovale is open, the flap being arranged so that most of the blood coming from below passes through it to the left atrium, left ventricle and so to the head and neck. In this way the best part of the supply from the mother goes to the coronary arteries and brain. Most of the blood from the superior vena cava and some of the blood from the inferior vena cava, passes through the tricuspid valve to the pulmonary artery. From here a little goes through the lungs, but most of it goes through the ductus arteriosus and down the aorta to the lower part of the body. The umbilical arteries take blood from the lower part of the body back to the placenta.

This arrangement ensures that the most vital structures, the brain and the heart, get the best of the oxygenated blood, and the blood returning to the placenta is that with the lowest oxygen saturation.

At birth the child fills its lungs with air and begins to cry. This puts up the pressure in the chest, and so raises the pressure in the left atrium, tending to close the foramen ovale. The great increase in blood returning from the lungs also fills the left atrium and so helps close the foramen ovale.

The blood circulates through the lungs at a lower pressure than the blood in the aorta. The ductus arteriosus is now connecting the aorta to a pulmonary artery in which the pressure has fallen. The flow of blood therefore reverses, and blood, fully oxygenated by the lungs, passes through the ductus arteriosus into the lungs. The ductus arteriosus is lined with muscle sensitive to this high oxygen tension. This muscle contracts when the oxygen tension rises and the ductus closes. The normal adult circulation is thus established, usually within a few minutes of birth.

2

Physiology of the heart

The heart is a muscular pump which needs oxygen and sugar for energy. These reach the muscle through the coronary arteries which supply a network of capillaries throughout the myocardium (the muscle of the heart). Carbon dioxide and other products of the heart work, such as pyruvic acid, are carried away by the blood in the capillaries to the venous blood, which passes through the lungs where the carbon dioxide is given up and fresh oxygen absorbed.

DISORDERED PHYSIOLOGY
Angina

It is fairly easy to get samples of venous blood from the heart muscle, by passing a cardiac catheter into the coronary sinus. Even in the heart of a normal resting subject, there is only about 25 per cent of the oxygen left in the blood after it has passed through the coronary arteries and veins to supply the muscle wall of the heart. In other words, the heart has used about three quarters of the available oxygen. In the muscles of the limbs, the blood gives up only about a quarter of the oxygen in its passage through them. This means that if the blood, for any reason, is carrying less oxygen than normal, the heart has very little reserve to fall back on and the heart muscle will suffer from lack of oxygen long before the limb muscles. Obvious causes of impairment of oxygen carrying capacity are anaemia or breathing air of a low oxygen content, as at high altitudes. A reduction in the cardiac output will have a similar effect. Breathlessness and eventually heart failure will occur as symptoms of this inadequate supply of oxygen to the heart, whether the cause is anaemia, mountain air, or the low output of heart disease.

To compensate for conditions such as anaemia or living at high altitudes, the quantity of blood flowing through the coronary arteries has to increase. It has been shown that in anaemia, the first compensation is the extraction of more of the oxygen from the blood passing through the heart muscle. Later (below a Hb of 50 per cent), the coronary flow must be increased. The heart must therefore work harder to pump this increased flow round, and it is not surprising that the heart muscle shows changes under the microscope indicating that it is suffering. When the oxygen supply is insufficient and the heart is driven too hard, the chemical change of the sugar to carbon dioxide becomes increasingly incomplete, leading to excessive production of such substances as pyruvates. These cause *pain in the muscle*. This usually makes the sufferer slow down or stop, and so reduces the rate at which the heart has to work. This allows the muscle to work more normally, the abnormal chemistry ceases, and with it the pain. This pain is called *angina* and is felt by the whole heart in anaemia or in mountaineers who exercise at high altitudes. Where an artery is narrowed by disease, the pain will occur in the part of the heart beyond the narrowed vessel.

Any muscle will have this pain if it is made to work with too little blood. You can easily produce it in your own arm by working the arm above your head. The pressure in the heart is only about two pounds per square inch (100 mm Hg). This is too low to supply enough blood to the arm above the head if it is working. For example, you will find that if you try to wash a ceiling you soon have to stop because your arm has become painful. When you rest the arm by your side the pain soon goes off and you can continue working. This is the same sort of pain as the pain in the chest due to heart ischaemia (lack of blood).

Valve leaks

When the valves in the heart leak, the chamber in the heart proximal to the leak (i.e. behind the leak) becomes over-loaded. When the mitral valve leaks, the atrium will receive during ventricular contraction (systole) the blood which leaks back, and at the same time will go on filling with the blood coming through from the lungs. To keep the blood going forward, more blood than normal will enter the ventricle during relaxation (diastole), so the stroke volume (the volume ejected at each beat) of the left ventricle is bigger than that of the right ventricle, if the right side is normal. This leads to enlargement of the left ventricle and a rise in pressure in the left atrium. The main symptom is breathlesness. Similarly, on the right side, tricuspid incompetence causes overfilling of the right atrium, a rise in right atrial pressure, and so engorgement of the veins of the neck. If the leak on the right side is considerable, the systolic reflux (back flow) into the right atrium will cause a systolic filling of the neck veins and congestion, enlargement, and systolic pulsation of the liver. In the liver this may lead to cirrhosis and, in some patients, to jaundice.

Leaking of the ventricular outflow valves (the aortic and pulmonary valves) has the same effect on ventricular stroke volume. Here the ventricle fills during diastole with blood entering normally from the atria, and it receives in addition the blood leaking back from the aorta or pulmonary artery. The arterial pulsation is therefore greater than normal, and, on the systemic side (the aorta and its branches), this is measurable as the increase in the pulse pressure, i.e. the difference between systolic and diastolic pressures. In severe aortic incompetence the blood pressure may be 140/40 mm Hg instead of the normal 120/80 mm Hg. The pulse pressure is 100 mm Hg instead of 40 mm Hg.

Valve narrowing

Narrowing of valve orifices is called *stenosis*. When this occurs the heart has to work harder to force the blood through the narrowed valve. The increased work makes the muscle of the chamber whose outflow is narrowed thicken. This is called *hypertrophy*. The narrowing may be enough to reduce the output of the heart. When this happens the patient develops symptoms due to the reduced output. Other symptoms, however, may be due to the increased pressure needed to force the blood through the narrow valves.

For example, in aortic stenosis, the symptoms are usually chest pain due to angina or fainting attacks, both the effect of the low output. Breathlessness is a late symptom because the mitral valve protects the lungs until late in the disease. In mitral stenosis, however, the pressure is felt first in the lung veins which become congested. This leads to oedema in the lungs and shortness of breath (dyspnoea) is the first symptom, although the output is reduced early. Fainting, however, is an unusual symptom in mitral stenosis.

Muscle damage

The muscle of the heart may be damaged by disease of the arteries or by conditions which affect the body as a whole. We have already mentioned anaemia, cyanosis and residence at high altitude. Other general conditions are thyrotoxicosis and myxoedema. It is perhaps to be expected that an overactive thyroid (thyrotoxicosis) should affect the heart, since the raised level of thyroid secretion acts like an accelerator on the metabolic rate, so that the heart has to go faster than normal. There seems to be some sort of particular action on the heart, since the increase in heart output in thyrotoxicosis is more than is strictly required for the increased metabolic rate. The heart enlarges, and in some patients the rhythm becomes irregular due to atrial fibrillation.

It is rather more surprising that myxoedema (underactive thyroid) is associated with heart change. A proportion of patients with myxoedema develop angina, with changes in the electrocardiogram. The angina clears up and the electrocardiogram reverts to normal when the disease is treated with thyroid preparations.

Other general conditions which affect the heart are those causing disturbances in blood electrolytes, particularly potassium and calcium. For example, severe diarrhoea with potassium depletion can cause serious cardiac disability.

Any generalized toxaemia may be associated with cardiac weakness. Severe pneumonia (particularly those due to staphylococci and Frielander's bacillus), virus infections, typhoid fever etc. can all be associated with myocardial damage.

Local damage to the heart is usually the result of coronary artery disease, where an artery is narrowed or blocked. Chest injury (particularly the stove-in chest of the car driver) and gun shot wounds are occasionally causes of local injury.

COMPENSATION FOR DAMAGE. Whatever the cause of cardiac muscle damage, the first response to compensate for the condition is the same. The muscle fibres can keep up their pressure by lengthening. It was shown many years ago, that the force with which a muscle contracts is proportional to its length—the further it is pulled out the more strongly it contracts. The heart's enlargement therefore compensates for its weakness. It usually does not empty as completely as normal, so that the volume in the ventricle at the end of systole (the *end-systolic volume*) is raised. The stroke volume may be reduced, in which case the output is maintained by an increase in heart rate, or the stroke volume may, in a less severely affected heart, be normal, in which case the rate may be normal at rest. Any exercise or infection, however, will usually cause a more rapid heart rate than normal in a patient with such a heart.

This lengthening of the muscle fibres in response to stress with consequent increased force of contraction, is called *Starling's Law* of the heart, after Sir Ernest Starling who first described it.

MAINTENANCE OF THE CIRCULATION

So far we have considered in a general way the heart as a pump, and discussed in outline some of the principles which govern its action in health and disease. We tend to think of the heart as a pump driving the blood round, rather in the same way as a pump drives the water round a central heating system in a house. There are, however, two fundamental differences between the circulation in the body and the circulation in a heating system. These are very important in understanding the nature of all sorts of events in the circulation and they underly the state called shock, in which the circulation fails because of a great fall in arterial pressure.

The first of these differences is the collapsible nature of the veins. This is common place knowledge: the veins on the back of your hand are full of blood when the hand is lying in your lap. When the hand is raised above the head, the blood runs down and the veins empty. This has one important effect. When anyone is lying horizontal, the heart has only to pump blood round the circulation which is all on one level. When they stand up, the blood pressure now has to raise blood up to the head because, as the veins collapse, there is no siphon effect which occurs in a rigid system like a central heating system. In a rigid system, the weight of the water coming down to the pump counterbalances the weight of water rising to the top of the system. We shall come back to how the body compensates for changes of this kind later.

The second difference is equally important. Apart from the slight differences due to temperature, a central heating system has a volume which can be measured and does not change. The vessels of the body, however, are much more complex. The large arteries are elastic, the small ones are very muscular, the capillaries have an enormous capacity and are never all open at the same time, and the veins have muscular walls and can vary their capacity.

Intelligent nursing of a patient with any circulatory disturbances, requires an understanding of the way in which the circulation is maintained. It will become evident that the heart plays a much smaller part in this than might be expected. We may start with the blood leaving the left ventricle and entering the aorta.

Arterial system

The pressure changes involved are shown in Fig.8. In diastole, blood enters the ventricle at a pressure of a little above zero. The ventricle then contracts and the pressure is suddenly raised to about 120 mm Hg. The aortic valve opens and about 70 ml blood is ejected into the aorta. The aorta is an elastic artery and swells up as the blood comes into it, the pressure quickly rising to 120 mm Hg. The aortic valve closes and the aorta gradually deflates, letting the pressure fall slowly until, by the time the next beat comes, the pressure is about 80 mm Hg. The closure of the valve causes a little jerk in the fall in pressure, called the dicrotic notch. If the artery becomes hardened and loses its elasticity, as happens in many old people, the cushioning effect is reduced, and the pressure may be as much as 190/90 mm Hg. This is a normal pressure for many people over 60 years old, and indicates not high blood pressure, but loss of elasticity of the arteries.

The blood flows through a series of branching arteries that become less elastic and more muscular as they get smaller. The final arteries

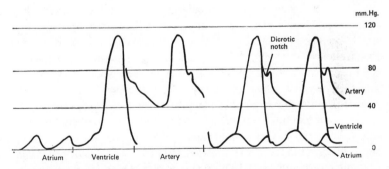

Fig.8. A diagram showing the typical pressure changes found in the normal heart. These changes have been traced from actual recordings taken on the left side of the heart. On the left of the diagram the pressure changes in the atrium, ventricle, and aorta are shown separately. On the right of the diagram they are combined to show the way in which the pressure is raised from 0 to arterial levels. In this patient, the rate with which the ventricular pressure rose and fell was rather slower than is normal, resulting in a much more cone shaped tracing than is often seen. The dicrotic notch is much exaggerated on the right hand side. This is often seen in patients who are being monitored. It is due to the elasticity of the recording tubing and is an exaggeration of the normal notch which occurs when the aortic valve closes.

are quite small and are called arterioles. They are normally held in a state of partial contraction (called tonus or tone), by a balance of impulses coming from the autonomic nerves, and chemicals circulating in the blood, some of which cause contraction and some relaxation. This balance is constantly being adjusted by circumstances causing changes either in the contraction or relaxation of the vessels. It is the *peripheral resistance* of these arterioles which ultimately maintains the blood pressure. Two examples of their action may be given here.

The first is a change concerned with the regulation of body temperature. When you are in a warm environment, the body needs to lose heat to prevent the body temperature rising. The rate of heat loss from the hands is increased by rise in the temperature of the hands. This is achieved by thousands of small arterioles in the palms and fingers, which open up and allow a great increase in blood flow. The temperature of the finger tips rises to about 36° C. Heat is lost from the hands by radiation and conduction. If you then go into the cold, the arterioles in the hand shut down and the hands become cold—about 2° C above the environmental temperature. If you then begin to make snowballs, the hands soon become red and rather painful. This is because the cold has reduced the circulation so much, that metabolic products of the tissues of the hands have not been carried away by the circulation, which is too slow for this to happen. These metabolic products make the vessels open up, the hands become red, and the metabolic products are carried away. In this sequence of events, the nervous control of the blood vessels in the fingers has first caused the arterioles to open when it was warm, and then to close when it was cold. Then a chemical stimulus has over-ridden the nervous control to protect the hands from frost-bite.

A second example was nicely demonstrated at the beginning of this century by a German Professor. He supported a man on a series of weighing machines, so that the arms, legs, head, chest and abdomen were all weighed separately while the man lay on his back. The man then ate a meal. The weights changed as blood was withdrawn from the limbs, which became lighter and was diverted to the abdomen, which became heavier. Blood was diverted to the abdomen to increase the blood supply to the gut, to enable digestion of the meal.

Capillaries

From the arterioles the blood enters the small vessels called capillaries.

These have very thin walls and are so narrow that the red blood cells have to push their way through. The walls, which are formed by a single layer of stretched out cells, allow substances in solution to pass freely through them, if the size of the molecule is small—for example, electrolytes like sodium and chloride. Large molecules like protein are less able to pass through the capillary wall and so come to create a force, tending to draw fluid back into the capillary. This is called colloid osmotic pressure (COP). There is a balance of pressures in the capillaries. At the arterial end, the blood pressure forces fluids out into the tissue spaces. This fluid takes with it oxygen, sugar, electrolytes etc. to nourish the tissues. At the venous end of the capillaries, the pressure in the vessels has fallen because the pressure has been dissipated in forcing the blood through the capillary. The COP of the blood now draws fluid back into the blood, this fluid bringing with it waste products like urea, and products of metabolism like pyruvates etc. Not all the fluid is drawn back—some finds its way back into the circulation as lymph.

The capillaries normally tend to close spontaneously. This is an effect of surface tension. The effect is similar to that acting on a new polythene bag. You have probably noticed that these are very difficult to open and tend to close themselves. Once the surface is dirty or crumpled, of course, this effect is lost. In the capillaries, just as in the bag, the sides are forced open if the pressure is high enough. We may imagine the normal capillary bed as consisting of a very large number of tiny tubes, mostly closed, with blood flowing through a few. If the tissue through which the vessels are passing increases its metabolic rate—for example, muscle starts working or gut digesting—the products of this metabolism act on the capillaries, causing more capillaries to open, and so increasing the flow. If very large numbers open up, the increased flow may be more than the heart and circulation can cope with and the blood pressure may fall. This may occur, for example, in someone who is badly burned, or in someone who has taken too much of a drug which causes the capillaries to dilate, tabs. Trinitrin or Amyl Nitrite for example.

Veins

From the capillaries the blood passes into a system of veins which, for the most part, run beside the corresponding arteries. (The veins of the brain, the liver, and the lungs are the chief exceptions.) The veins have muscular walls and, at intervals, have valves, which allow

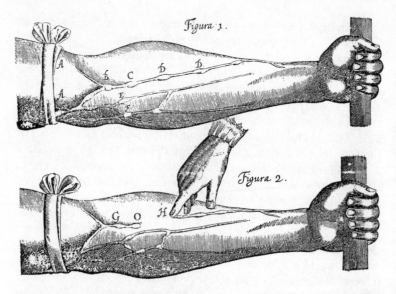

Fig.9. An illustration from Harvey's book on the circulation of the blood. It shows in the upper figure a man's arm with a tourniquet on. The veins are distended and the valves are marked by letters. In the lower picture the blood has been emptied out of the section shown between C and D by placing a finger to close the vein at D. The blood is then milked out of the section up to the valve C, and as shown in the lower figure, it does not refill. If the finger at H is now lifted the section of vein fills immediately because the valve D allows blood to pass up towards the shoulder.

blood to pass back towards the heart but not to return towards the periphery. Their action is easily demonstrated with two fingers on the veins of the forearm or back of the hand. In showing this non-return action we are repeating the experiment of Harvey, who described the circulation of the blood about 200 years ago (Fig.9).

As well as returning blood to the heart, veins have another important function—they act as a reservoir for blood. This action of the veins was clearly shown by observations made on blood donors. X-rays were taken of the chest before and after the donors had given a pint of blood. The x-rays showed that after bleeding the lung veins were thinner than they had been before. The donors' venous pressure had been maintained by the muscles in the vein walls contracting to take up the slack in the circulation caused by the loss of a pint of blood.

Adjustment to change in posture

We may now consider a simple example of how the circulation adapts itself to a change in its equilibrium, by describing in outline the readjustments needed when someone gets out of bed.

While lying flat the blood is pumped round in the circulation fairly easily. All the arteries are more or less at the same level, and the blood is returned to the heart from the great veins, largely by the pumping action of the chest wall. As the chest is expanded, the elastic lungs are pulled out to fill them with air and this suction causes a small negative pressure (of a few cm water) in the chest. This sucks blood into the right atrium, so that the filling of the right side of the heart is better during inspiration than expiration. In an average adult man, the output of the heart is about 5 litres per minute in this position.

On standing erect, the first thing that happens is that the blood fills up the veins in the lower part of the body. This causes a fall in the return of blood to the right atrium of about 1 litre per minute, and so a fall in the output of the heart (CO) to about 4 litres per minute. Without some adjustment, this fall in output would cause a fall in blood pressure.

Two other events occur which tend to cause a fall in blood pressure. The first is the change in the position of the head relative to the heart. When the body is horizontal, the pump (the heart) is on the same level as the head, so the normal blood pressure (mean pressure about 100 mm Hg or two pounds per square inch) is easily able to push blood along to the head. When erect, the blood has now to be lifted to the head which is 30 or 40 cm above the heart.

The third factor which affects the blood pressure is the peripheral resistance in the arterioles. When the body is horizontal all the blood vessels are more or less at the same level, so gravity has little effect. When the body is standing, the vessels of the feet are exposed to the pressure at which the blood is pumped from the heart, plus the weight of the column of blood between the heart and the feet. Similarly the pressure in the vessels of the head, is the pumping pressure of the heart *minus* the weight of blood between the heart and the head. Any nurse who has learned how to take the blood pressure with a sphygmomanometer, can easily confirm this phenomenon. First measure the blood pressure carefully with the arm at the patient's side. Then raise the arm above the patient's head, keeping the patient's position otherwise unaltered. The pressure in the arm with the arm raised, is about 20–30 mm Hg lower than when the arm is down.

Clearly all these factors will tend to make the blood pressure fall, particularly in the highest part of the circulation, the head. Equally, the circulation cannot anticipate these changes, and can only react to them after they have occurred, or as they are occurring. The maintenance of a constant pressure in the blood supply to the head is essential to consciousness and is primarily due to pressure receptors in the carotid sinuses. The carotid sinuses are two bulges—one in each of the carotid arteries—where they divide in the neck at the level of the angle of the jaw, i.e. the level of the base of the skull. When the pressure falls in the carotid sinuses, they immediately send nervous impulses up to the brain, where the main centre controlling the circulatory system is located in the medulla oblongata. The tonus (resistance) of the peripheral arterioles all over the body is readjusted, to increase the resistance to the flow of blood in arteries below the heart and to maintain pressure and flow to the brain. In addition, the heart rate is usually increased.

This readjustment may take up to 15 seconds to be complete, and until the readjustments are effective the person who has stood up may feel rather dizzy. If they are unaccustomed to standing (like a patient who has been very ill and nursed flat), they may faint. If the circulation is already committed to a considerable degree, for example, in a hot environment, to pumping a lot of blood through the skin for cooling purposes, the dizziness may be severe and last longer. People getting out of a hot bath or lifting something from a hot oven may have noticed this.

Standing still by the bed with the circulation adjusted, the pressure in the ankle veins is the same as a column of blood reaching up to the right atrium—120 cm or so, and the output of the heart (the same as the venous return) is about 20 per cent less than that when recumbent. If the subject now began to walk, the pressure in the ankle veins falls to about 40 cm as the muscles of the legs pump blood back up the veins of the legs. This is achieved because the valves in the veins only allow the blood to move up towards the heart. When the veins are squeezed by the muscles, therefore, the blood is pumped up to beyond the valves, and on the muscle relaxing, the vein refills from below. This increased return of venous blood, of course, means an increased cardiac output. Postural dizziness, therefore, is something which occurs when the subject is standing still. It is virtually unknown in someone who is walking about.

We have considered this simple change of position in some detail as it is of great importance in nursing. We now turn from the working of the healthy heart to consider disease. To do this we must accept a difficulty. Many factors can cause heart disease but the result of these processes is a common one—heart failure. Some of these factors have already been mentioned. We shall now consider how the heart may fail, and what the effects of this failure are. When later we encounter the various heart diseases, we will be able to discuss the failure of the heart with some idea of what this means. This seems a more helpful way of tackling the problems of heart disease, than to describe the heart diseases first and the failure afterwards. For the next chapter, therefore, we will consider heart failure as it might arise in any one of several diseases.

3

Heart failure

Heart failure is a disorder of the function of the heart. The normal heart has a large reserve of power which allows it to increase its output about three times during exercise without distress. When its normal function is disturbed by disease, it can draw upon this capacity to maintain its output without failing. This available capacity is called the *cardiac reserve*. Eventually if the disturbance of function due to disease progresses far enough, the heart can no longer maintain the output and the pressure in the veins returning blood to the heart will rise. This rise in venous pressure is the earliest sign of heart failure.

The work of the heart is primarily to raise the pressure in the ventricle from zero to about 30 mm Hg on the right side, and to 120 mm Hg on the left side. The first effect of the rise in pressure in the atrium due to heart failure, is to reduce the gradient between the atrium concerned and the great artery into which the blood is being pumped.

LEFT HEART FAILURE

This rise in pressure is, in fact, a late compensation for disordered function. We may now consider the stages of the heart's compensation and failure.

1. *Enlargement of the left ventricle.* If there is a posterior coronary thrombosis which mainly affects the left ventricle, the initial compensation of the heart to the infarct (the dead muscle), is to enlarge the left ventricle slightly and so increase the force of the contraction by the remaining healthy muscle (Starling's Law). This will maintain the output, but, as the volume of the ventricle will be increased, and the stroke volume unchanged, the ventricle will not empty as

completely as normal. This means that both the end diastolic volume (the volume in the ventricle at the end of its filling phase) and the end systolic volume (the volume in the ventricle at the end of the contraction) will be bigger than normal (usually termed 'raised').

2. *Increase in heart rate.* In a larger infarct, the next compensation will be an increase in rate of the heart by perhaps 20 or 30 beats a minute. This helps the heart by reducing the stroke volume.

3. *Fall in ventricular output.* If the heart is even more severely affected, the left ventricular output may fall. Blood returning to the right side of the heart will be pumped normally into the lungs and will begin to accumulate in the pulmonary veins. The left ventricle is now failing.

4. *Increase in left atrial pressure.* The pressure in these pulmonary veins will now rise and so will the pressure in the left atrium. This will mean that the left ventricle has less work to do—for example, suppose the left atrial pressure rises from a mean of 3 mm Hg to a mean of 13 mm Hg. The ventricle will now have to increase the blood pressure from 13 to 120 mm Hg instead of from 3 to 120 mm Hg, i.e. by about 107 mm Hg instead of by 117 mm Hg. This it may well be able to do and, if the condition is a stable one (i.e. the heart is not getting better or worse), the patient will be able to get about and do a light job. He will find, however, that if he does anything involving more exertion than usual, such as climbing a flight of stairs, the increased venous return from the muscles when pumped through the lungs is too much for the left ventricle. The left atrial pressure rises further, and he has either to stop at the top of the stairs 'to get his breath back' while the inefficient ventricle clears the blood from the lungs, or he can manage to carry on if he goes up slowly—thereby keeping the increase in venous return down to a level the left ventricle can deal with. This state of affairs, which may be found in the right side or the left side or both sides of the heart simultaneously, is usually called *compensated heart failure.* The cardiac output is maintained at normal limits at rest, but on exertion the output does not rise to the heights that it should and a temporary further increase in venous pressure occurs.

5. *Development of pulmonary oedema.* Should things get worse in this patient, the pressure will rise further in the left atrium, until the venous pressure in the lungs exceeds the colloid osmotic pressure (COP) of the blood (see page 19). When this happens the normal circulation in the capillaries is disturbed, as the pressure of the left

atrium and pulmonary veins is transmitted back to the venous side of the capillaries. Fluid will leave the capillaries on the arterial side in the normal way but be unable to re-enter the vessels on the venous side. It will therefore remain in the tissues of the lung as oedema fluid. The normal COP of plasma is about 25 mm Hg and the tissue COP about 10 mm Hg. If the left atrial pressure rises to 20 mm Hg it would appear that the fluid must continue to pass into the tissue spaces of the lung until the patient has died of pulmonary oedema. In practice the left atrial pressure can be consistently over 25 mm Hg in conditions like mitral stenosis, where the rise in pressure is due to the obstruction of the narrowed mitral valve. We must now digress to see how this comes about.

It is a common observation that many patients with heart disease cannot lie flat without getting very distressed and short of breath. If they slip down off their pillows in sleep, they waken very dyspnoeic and have to sit on the edge of the bed for perhaps as long as half an hour or more before feeling well enough to lie on their pillows again. (This inability to lie flat is called *orthopnoea* and the awakening dyspnoea at night is called *paroxysmal nocturnal dyspnoea*).

These are people who have a high left atrial pressure. Just as in the systemic circulation the pressure in an artery is the resultant of the pressure generated in the heart and the distance above or below the heart, falling as the distance rises above the heart and rising as the distance falls below the heart, so it is in the veins of the lungs. In the pulmonary veins the pressure will be all fairly similar with the patient lying flat, as the distance between the lung vessels in the front and at the back is only 10–15 cm, equivalent to about 10 mm Hg. If the left atrial pressure is 30 mm Hg the difference will be about 25 mm Hg for the front to 35 mm Hg for the back. When erect, the lungs are about 40 cm from top to bottom (or apex to base to be more technical). This is equivalent to about 30 mm Hg with the left atrium about half way up. This means that with the patient sitting up, the pressure in the veins at the bases is about 45 mm Hg in our patient, but at the apex is only 15 mm Hg. When lying flat generalized pulmonary oedema will develop. Sitting up, the bases of the lungs will be oedematous but the apices will be clear.

If the transudation of fluid due to the higher pressure continues, it will begin to pass through into the alveoli producing crepitations (fine moist sounds) as the wet surfaces separate when air is drawn into them by breathing. This condition will progress to one where there is enough fluid to be coughed up. Such sputum is usually rather watery, frothy, and in severe acute cases, often tinged with blood.

6a. *Peripheral cyanosis.* Further downward progress is usually marked by cyanosis. This may be peripheral due to slowing of the circulation. The blood circulates more slowly because the output is reduced and so the blood passes through the capillaries more slowly and is more completely depleted of oxygen than usual. This causes blueness of the lips and cheeks and is known as peripheral cyanosis. Similar slowing with blueness occurs if the skin is cold.

6b. *Central cyanosis.* The fluid accumulating in the tissue spaces of the lungs slows up the transfer of gases between the alveoli and the capillaries. As a result blood may pass through the alveoli without picking up its full amount of oxygen. The arterial blood leaving the left heart will then not be fully oxygenated. This results in central cyanosis evident in blueness of the tongue as well as of the lips and cheeks.

The appearance of peripheral cyanosis in heart failure, provided the patient is warm, indicates a serious drop in heart output. Central cyanosis in a previously normally coloured patient usually means that serious pulmonary oedema is present. Central cyanosis in acute heart failure is very important, as the heart is very sensitive to anything which reduces the quantity of oxygen in blood (see page 12), and the appearance of central cyanosis due to heart failure will further depress the heart action.

7. *Death.* Finally, if the failure of the left ventricle continues the patient dies of left heart failure, progressive pulmonary oedema gradually reducing the oxygen in the blood and so the heart's capacity to contract. The progress from normal to death from pulmonary oedema, may take five minutes or many years depending on how the heart is affected by the infarct.

This progression of events in the failure of the left heart has been described in detail because it is important, and because it may not be very obvious looking at the patient. The clinical picture in its early stages is of dyspnoea on effort. Later the patient is orthopnoeic and usually has a tachycardia. Later still the patient begins to bring up frothy sputum which may be tinged with blood. Finally the patient is usually cold, cyanosed and unconscious. We cannot easily measure the pressure in the left atrium and pulmonary veins. We can only see their effects. A chest x-ray, however, will usually show the typical appearances of pulmonary oedema and allow a usually reliable assessment of whether the changes are acute or chronic.

RIGHT HEART FAILURE

Failure of the right side of the heart follows a similar pattern to that on the left, but as the veins concerned are visible, it is much easier to appreciate its results. The stages of enlargement and tachycardia to compensate for early damage, are often not appreciated by the patient.

1. *Increase in venous pressure.* The first obvious sign of the right heart's inability to cope with its load, is elevation of the pressure in the external jugular veins. These veins are easily seen in the neck and are usually a reliable gauge of the systemic venous pressure. The elevation of pressure in the veins, however, should be present when the patient is lying quietly propped up at 45°, for venous pressure in the neck depends both on the position of the body and the pressure in the thorax. The jugular veins fill in most people if they lie flat, as the veins then lie below the level of the right atrium. They also fill if the thoracic pressure is raised by coughing or talking. Watch the neck of anyone who speaks continuously for more than a few seconds. As the flow of words continues, the veins fill and the level of the top of the venous column rises until they stop speaking. On drawing breath, the veins collapse dramatically as the pressure in the thorax changes from positive to negative. Other things may cause a distension of neck veins—pressure from a collar, pressure from glands in the thoracic inlet, scarring from an injury or radiotherapy or obstruction by thrombosis.

2. *Oedema of the tissues.* Increased venous pressure leads to oedema of the tissues in the same way as in left heart failure. Here it is related to position and, just as in the lung, is found in the dependent parts. The patient suffering from right heart failure, therefore, notices oedema in the feet in the evening, which disappears during the night. Later the swelling may be present all day, and spread up the body to the abdomen or backs of the hands. The high venous pressure, if prolonged, causes liver enlargement, enlargement of the spleen and a poor circulation through the gut leading to poor digestion, much wind in the gut, and a poor secretion of urine, as the filtration by the kidney is upset both by the change in pressure and by the slowing of the circulation.

3. *Tricuspid incompetence.* The tricuspid valve, it has been said

earlier (page 8) is not very efficient. It becomes incompetent easily in dilatation of the right ventricle. When the ventricle contracts against an incompetent valve, some of the contents are driven back into the right atrium, causing a large pulse to pass up the neck (the 'V' wave). The pulsation is also transmitted to the liver which may become tense and painful.

4. *Liver and renal failure.* If the failure gets worse the patient may show liver failure (jaundice) or renal failure (oliguria with concentrated urine). Less commonly, the oedema spreads up to involve the chest and arms.

Long continuous failure leads to permanent enlargement of the liver and a form of cirrhosis.

FAILURE DUE TO ABNORMAL RATE

A healthy heart may fail if it goes too fast or too slow for long periods. The way in which these disturbances of rhythm embarrass the heart are important to our understanding of the treatment of heart failure, as tachycardia (rapid heart rate) or bradycardia (slow heart rate) frequently accompany failure from other causes.

Tachycardia

This may be due to many causes. The different causes of tachycardia will be considered later. Whatever the cause of the increase in heart rate, it has similar effects. As the heart rate rises to twice or three times normal, the output of the heart falls. The reason for this is the inability of the heart to increase its filling by suction on the part of the ventricles. When the heart rate increases in exercise, the tachycardia is a response to the increased venous return coming from the exercising muscles, and is accompanied by an increase in cardiac output—the venous return is normally the same as the cardiac output (see page 21). When the rate rises to 150 or 250 beats a minute in the resting patient, the time available for filling of the heart becomes shorter and shorter. As there is less and less time for the heart to fill, there is less and less blood for it to put out. In a patient who developed a heart rate of 190 during cardiac catheterization, the cardiac output fell to a quarter of normal.

A patient who suffers from attacks of paroxysmal tachycardia (bouts of rapid heart rate), is usually aware of the 'fluttering' in the chest. If the attack lasts more than a minute or two, a constricting chest pain comes on—angina pectoris—due to the effect of the low output on coronary flow. If the attack lasts for longer, heart failure with lung congestion, and a rise in the jugular venous pressure with, eventually, peripheral oedema develop. This usually takes several days. Restoration of a normal heart rate results in a gradual clearance of the congestion taking minutes, hours, or days, depending on the severity of the disturbances due to the tachycardia.

Bradycardia

This is a less obvious cause of embarrassment to the heart. When a heart beats at 30 or 40 beats a minutes, the patient has usually a reduced capacity to exercise and may suffer from heart failure. Attacks of unconsciousness due to abnormal rhythms may occur (Adams-Stokes attacks). The cause of this heart disability is a fall in the quantity of blood flowing through the coronary arteries, which occurs when the heart rate is very slow. During the long diastole in severe bradycardia, the diastolic pressure falls too low to perfuse the coronary arteries. This means that the coronary arteries only pass blood during early diastole, and no blood flows through the heart muscle during late diastole and systole. Speeding up the heart rapidly relieves the symptoms.

TREATMENT OF HEART FAILURE

With a knowledge of the working of the heart and an appreciation of the way in which it fails, it is possible, briefly, to consider the principles which underlie the treatment of heart failure. This treatment will be familiar to every nurse, and it is important to appreciate that it is largely treatment directed to putting right the effects of heart failure. Most of the measures considered are not directly treating the heart. The principles of treatment may be considered as follows:

Rest forms the basis of the treatment of heart failure. The position in which the patient is nursed depends upon the circumstances. If the patient's systemic blood pressure is low, the patient is best nursed flat or with the head down, as raising the head will lower the arterial pressure in the head. When the patient is suffering from pulmonary congestion, as in mitral valve stenosis, the patient is best nursed sitting up and may be best able to use the lungs if nursed seated in a cardiac chair.

Pain is exhausting and keeps patients awake. It is usually severe and may need the injection of an analgesic to relieve it.

Oxygen given by a nasal tube or oxygen tent will assist many patients with heart failure. A high oxygen tension will raise the oxygen content of the alveoli and so improve the transference of oxygen from the alveoli to the blood. It will have little effect in patients in whom the failure is confined to the right side of the heart, unless the lungs in these patients are diseased so causing cyanosis.

Diuretics, by increasing water loss from the kidneys, will diminish the total amount of water in the body. In failure of the left side of the heart, the fluid accumulating in the lungs will be diminished. Similarly in right heart failure, the oedema in the dependent parts of the body will be excreted.

Hypotension (low blood pressure) may be due to a variety of causes, for example poor ventricular contraction which may respond to drugs which stimulate the heart, and poor peripheral resistance due to loss of arterial tone, which may also respond to the appropriate drugs. A low blood pressure may also be due to a heart rate which is too high or too low.

Tachycardia may need to be controlled. Often this can be done by suitable drugs. Sometimes the abnormal rhythm will respond to electrical treatment. The purpose of this treatment is to slow the heart to give it time to fill and to allow the output to increase.

Bradycardia (slow heart rate) may also require treatment. Suitable drugs will often do this successfully. In some types of bradycardia, electrical stimulation of the heart may be needed (pacing).

4

The electrocardiogram

The electrocardiogram is the key to understanding disorders of heart rhythm. The electrocardiogram (ECG) has been known for about 100 years, having been first recorded by a Doctor Waller on his pet bulldog. The principle is a simple one. When any muscle contracts, it does so by the shortening of protein molecule chains within the cell. The energy used and the reaction itself are chemical. The change however, is accompanied by a movement of potassium ions from outside the cell wall to inside the cell wall. Since potassium (K^+) carries a positive charge, the contraction is accompanied by a change in voltage of the cell surface, from positive to negative. The electrocardiograph (the name given to the machine which records the electrocardiogram) is simply a sensitive voltmeter capable of recording millivolts (thousandths of volts). It is important to remember that all muscles have this property and so, if the ECG is being recorded from the limbs, movement or limb muscle tremor will also be recorded and produce voltage changes in the ECG.

THE NORMAL HEART BEAT

The normal heart beat starts up near the top of the right atrium in the sino-atrial node (SA node) and spreads across the atria. The SA node has the property of generating the heart beat and is affected by nervous control from the sympathetic and para-sympathetic (vagus) nerves. It is also affected by circulating hormones like adrenalin and by drugs. For example, if a normal person gets a shock —a sudden noise, or sudden bad news—their heart rate increases as a result of three effects. The sympathetic stimulation by nerves increases, the vagus tone (slowing) is diminished, and adrenalin may be released from the suprarenal glands. All these increase heart rate.

The beat next reaches the atrio-ventricular node at the bottom of the atrium. This starts an impulse which spreads down along the nervous pathway into the ventricles. This pathway is a nerve bundle called the bundle of His. This soon divides into two bundles of nerves which run down in the muscle of the septum between the ventricles, one in the right ventricle, one in the left. These bundles send out branches as they go, so that the beat is carried quickly to all parts of the ventricle. The contraction is completed by the change from 'resting' to 'contract', spreading from one cell to the next until all the cells are contracting. The change in voltage which accompanies this contraction is tiny for a single cell, but, for the whole heart, is enough to record on the ECG. It is roughly quantitative, for example it is more for the left ventricle than for the right—as the left ventricle is thicker than the right. After contracting the muscle relaxes to fill once more. For a short period the muscle is unable to contract even if it is stimulated. This is called the *refractory period*. After this it is once again able to contract.

The ECG is conventionally recorded from connections made to the limbs. This is because the early electrocardiographs were not very sensitive and needed a large area of skin contact for a satisfactory recording. Patients sat with their hands and feet in bowls of warm saline to which the machine was connected. The result was to make a triangle of possible connections—arm to arm and either arm to the leg. This is called Einthoven's triangle. Although this is not a very sensible way to analyse in two planes changes which are occurring in three planes (the heart), it is still the basis of the standard recording, as the variations of the voltages recorded are so well understood. Modern ECG machines are sensitive enough to record from a needle point if necessary, and an ECG can be recorded from any two points over the surface of the heart. The top and bottom of the sternum gives a very useful ECG with little chance of muscle movement interfering with the record.

THE NORMAL ECG

The normal ECG consists of a series of voltage changes resulting from the contraction of the atria and the contraction and recovery of the ventricles. The recovery of the atria does not usually cause a measurable change in the record (Fig.10). The direction of the voltage change is positive upwards and negative downwards from

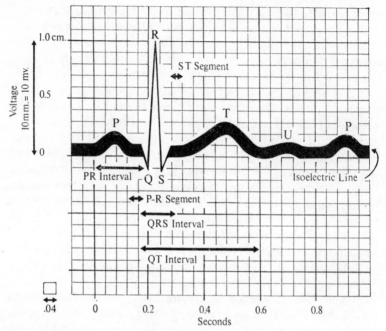

Fig.10. Diagram of the normal electrocardiogram shown on standard recording paper. The distance between each thick line horizontally represents 0·2 seconds at the standard rate of 25 mm per second and when correctly standardized each cm in a vertical direction is equivalent of 10 mv.

the O voltage line (called the iso-electric line). The main changes (usually called deflections) are given letters to identify them.

The first deflection is a small one due to the atrial contraction and is called the P wave. It is positive in most connections, and, when the machine is correctly adjusted (see page 124) is normally less than 3 mm high in the standard leads.

After a short return to the iso-electric line during which the contraction stimulus is passing through the AV node and bundle of His, the ventricle contracts. This produces the largest voltage swings, usually three. There is a brief downward (negative) swing, the Q wave, then a large upward swing, the R wave and then a further swing below to negative, the S wave. In some recordings the Q wave is absent, and in some the S wave is the largest. Sometimes these swings are repeated, and the second R and S waves are written R′ and S′. The voltage then returns to zero, the contraction completed. This group of movements is usually called the QRS complex. There then occurs a low upward deflection, the T wave, which indicates recovery. Some people have a small further upward swing, the U wave. The voltage becomes zero once more until the next beat occurs.

The timing of these events is important as prolongation of the conduction through the heart is found in certain diseases. The conduction time depends to some extent on the heart rate, and, naturally, on the size of the heart. Here we may consider the usual normal findings of an average sized adult, with a normal heart rate.

The interval between the beginning of the atrial beat and the beginning of the ventricular beat is called the *P-R interval*—or P-Q interval if the initial deflection of the ventricular complex is a Q wave. It is measured from the beginning of the deflection of the P wave from the iso-electric line to the first deviation from O of the QRS complex (see Fig.10). It should not exceed 0·2 seconds (5 mm of paper at normal recording speed), but may be as short as 0·12 seconds.

The QRS interval is the time taken for the beat to spread through the ventricles. This is normally not more than 0·1 seconds (half the P-R interval).

Two more features of the normal ECG must be noted. The first is the part of the tracing between the completion of the P wave and the beginning of the QRS complex. This is called the P-R segment. It is usually iso-electric and is rarely of critical importance. The other is the part of the tracing between the end of the QRS complex and the beginning of the T wave. This is the *S-T segment*. It is usually within a millimetre or two of the iso-electric line and is of very great importance. Deviations of this part of the tracing away from normal limits, usually indicate serious trouble.

5

Disorders of rhythm

Normal rhythm is usually called *sinus rhythm* as it originates in the sino-atrial node. Disorders of rhythm are usually called arrhythmias. Their importance to the patient depends on their effect upon the performance of the heart as a pump. This is simply that they make the heart go too fast (see page 29), too slow (see page 30) or stop. Many are of little clinical importance, but it is important to be familiar with their appearance as they may be mistaken for serious conditions. *Sinus arrhythmia* is a common finding in children but is uncommon in adults. In this condition the rate is irregular, being alternatively faster and slower. The alteration is usually a regular one in time with respiration. It is a normal phenomenon (Fig.11).

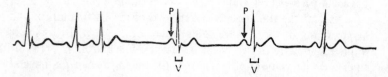

Fig.11. A normal electrocardiogram from a child showing sinus arrhythmia P indicates the P wave and V the QRS complex.

TACHYCARDIAS

Tachycardia means rapid heart rate. They are important as a cause of distressing symptoms and also because they may complicate the management of heart disease. All of them may occur in patients who have otherwise healthy hearts. They may also occur in patients with rheumatic heart disease and congenital heart disease. Other causes are drugs, where they may indicate overdosage or sensitivity in the patients. They are also found in electrolyte disturbances. They can be serious and sometimes fatal complications after coronary thrombosis or operations on the heart. The increasing use of monitoring oscilloscopes in general wards, means that nurses should be familiar with the appearance of the ECG of the commoner ones.

Atrial fibrillation

Atrial fibrillation is a common *cause of tachycardia* (Fig.12). In fibrillation the orderly spread of a contraction across the atrium ceases. Individual muscle cells continue to contract, however, but instead of the normal contraction and relaxation of the heart

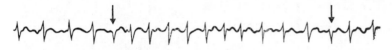

Fig.12. Uncontrolled atrial fibrillation. The heart rate is quite irregular and the iso-electric line shows an irregular variation. In this patient there are two complexes marked with arrows which appear to be extra systoles since the QRS complex is unlike the remainder.

chambers concerned, there is an erratic movement of contraction all over the muscle of the affected chambers. This causes no change in volume, and so there is no effective contraction. The atria have a striking appearance in this condition and appear to shimmer under the lights of the operating theatre.

The atrio-ventricular node is stimulated by the contracting muscle cells, often at a rate of 300 to 400 per minute. These rates are far beyond the capacity of the ventricle to respond to. As a result the ventricle is constantly being excited. As soon as the refractory period has passed the stimulus to contract is again received. As atrial fibrillation is common in patients with rheumatic heart disease where the valves may be diseased (see page 66) or the muscle weak (see page 66), severe heart failure commonly results.

Treatment

Treatment consists in slowing the heart. The most effective method is to restore sinus rhythm. This can often be done by passing an electric shock through the heart. This stops the heart completely and it will usually start up again spontaneously in sinus rhythm. The instrument used is a defibrillator (see page 93) coupled to an ECG so that the electric shock comes in the refractory period of the ventricle (just after the R wave). This coupling to the R wave is needed because an electric shock at the wrong time (e.g. on the T wave) is likely to make the ventricles fibrillate—and then the whole heart output stops.

Alternatively the heart can be slowed by drugs, the fibrillation persisting. The main drug used is digitalis (the leaf of the common purple foxglove, digitalis purpura) or one of its many preparations such as digoxin. These work by making it more difficult for impulses to pass down the atrio-ventricular node and the ventricular conducting system. As a result fewer of the impulses reaching the AV node are transmitted to the ventricular muscle and the rate slows (Fig.13).

ECTOPIC BEATS

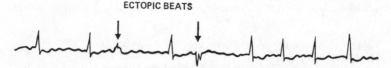

Fig.13. Atrial fibrillation slowed by digitalis. The rate is so regular that it could be easily missed by someone recording the pulse. The absence of the P waves on the electrocardiogram however, makes it easily recognized.

It is important to appreciate that the contribution of the atrial contractions to the cardiac output is small. The essential thing in treatment is to slow the rate, not to restore sinus rhythm. When once an atrium has fibrillated because of disease, it is likely to do so again, so to try to treat patients with atrial fibrillation by electrical defibrillation is usually unsuccessful, as the arrhythmias recur after seconds, days or months. The foxglove preparations are much more helpful—the only common symptom due to them in therapeutic doses being a loss of appetite.

Because of the irregular rate in atrial fibrillation, the beats of the ventricles vary in their size. When a long diastole has occurred, the heart has filled well and the systole will produce a large pulse in the arteries. When diastole has been short, the heart will have had little time to fill and the volume ejected during systole will be small. Consequently the pulse from that beat will be small. The blood pressure recorded under these circumstances will vary from beat to beat and, in rapid uncontrolled atrial fibrillation, many beats will be so small that they will not be felt at the wrist at all. This is made use of clinically by charting the rate at the apex of the heart, recorded by listening to the heart beats with a stethoscope, and *simultaneously* counting the rate at the wrist. The difference is a measure of the control of the heart action by treatment. When this is poor there will be many beats missing at the wrist. When it is good all will be detected. Obviously a simple chart of the heart rate (**not** the pulse) will do just as well as a measure of the success of treatment.

EXTRASYSTOLES

Extrasystoles are beats which originate in parts of the heart outside the normal pace maker (sino-atrial node). The word 'extra' means outside in Latin. They may start in the atria when they are called atrial extrasystoles, in the atrio-ventricular conducting system, when they are called nodal extrasystoles, or in the ventricles, when they are called ventricular extrasystoles. Everybody gets beats of this kind now and again, but most people are quite unaware of them.

They occur before the normal sinus beat should occur. The normal beat is then suppressed because it occurs while the heart is still refractory as a result of the extrasystole. The normal rhythm is then resumed, one normal beat having been missed. Because of the timing of the beats, the extrasystole causes a smaller pulse than normal, but the normally timed beat which follows the extrasystole is larger than normal because the heart has had longer to fill. It is often noticed by the patient as a bumping feeling, usually in the chest (Fig.14). Not infrequently, several extrasystoles will occur in short succession and the patient will notice a 'fluttering' sensation in the chest. These are often noticed when the patient is sitting still or is in bed. If they occur when the patient is busy they are often unnoticed. (Fig.15).

Paroxysmal tachycardia

Some patients get continuous runs of extrasystoles lasting minutes or hours. These attacks usually start suddenly and often stop as suddenly. The heart is usually normal apart from this unfortunate tendency to bouts of tachycardia. The condition is called paroxysmal tachycardia and the symptoms depend upon the rate of the heart and the duration of the attack, ranging from merely an uncomfortable fluttering in the chest, to severe anginal pain with a sensation of impending death called anguor amini. If an attack lasts several hours, heart failure may occur.

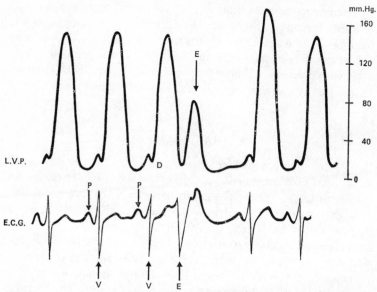

Fig.14. A recording taken at cardiac catheterization showing the left ventricular pressure and the electrocardiogram. The left ventricular pressure is about 160/0, the P waves are rather large, and there is an obvious A wave in the pressure tracing due to the forceful contraction of the atrium. The patient had aortic stenosis and the rather conical pressure tracings are due to the thickened ventricle. The P waves are shown by the letter P, the QRS complexes by V. At E an extra systole occurs and the ventricular beat corresponding to this is much smaller as the ventricle has had little time to fill. The normal beat occurring next after the extra systole, is larger than normal owing to the longer time the ventricle has had to fill. Note that the electrical changes occur a little in advance of the pressure changes. This is a normal finding. The slight dip in the tracing after the A wave lettered D on the pressure tracing, is a false appearance due to the elasticity of the cardiac catheter through which the tracing was made. In reality the pressure increases steadily from the peak of the A wave into the rise due to ventricular contraction. On the right the pressures are shown. Normally the lines indicating the pressure are continued across the pressure tracing but have been omitted in the diagram for the sake of simplicity.

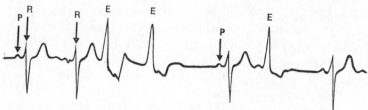

Fig.15. A tracing showing ventricular extra systoles. P P-wave, R R-wave, E extra systole. Note that two P waves could not be identified as they coincide with the V wave of the extra systole.

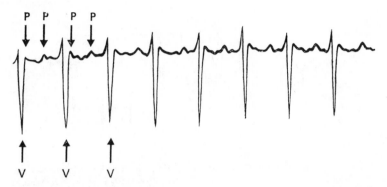

Fig.16. Atrial tachycardia with two to one block. P P-wave, V V-wave. Note that every other P wave occurs when the ventricle is refractory and does not result in a ventricular contraction.

The rhythm is usually the same in any patient in all their attacks.

Atrial tachycardia is commonly found with a varying amount of block. For example, the atrial rate in such an attack is often a regular beat of 300 a minute. Usually the ventricle is only able to respond to every other beat of the atrium, so a regular pulse rate of 150 a minute results (Fig.16). This is called 2:1 block—2 atrial to 1 ventricular beat.

In some patients the degree of block is greater or less and the ventricle may respond to 2 out of 3 atrial beats or to only one in three. Sometimes the degree of block varies continuously, giving an irregular pulse like that of atrial fibrillation (Fig.17).

Nodal tachycardia may occur less commonly. In many cases the exact site of the focus causing the arrhythmia cannot be decided with certainty. When it is evidently originating from somewhere above the ventricles, the term *supraventricular tachycardia* is often used to describe it.

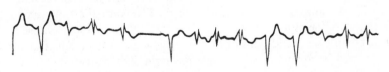

Fig.17. A grossly irregular tracing showing extra systoles arising in several different places in the heart (multi-focal extra systoles) some with a dominant S wave and some with a dominant R wave.

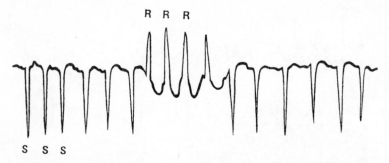

Fig.18. Ventricular tachycardia. In this tracing the main deflection is an S wave, the RS and T are marked. The P waves could not be clearly identified. The rate is regular and very rapid. Four beats lettered R originate in a different part of the heart.

Ventricular tachycardia. In ventricular tachycardia the heart is driven by an ectopic focus in the ventricle itself (Fig.18). The rhythm is usually regular and is particularly likely to cause syncope heart failure. This is because the ventricle is directly stimulated and so maintains the rate set by the abnormal irritable focus which has taken over the pacing of the ventricle.

These rhythms are all important. They will be referred to again as the various conditions in which they occur are encountered.

BRADYCARDIA

Bradycardia means slow heart beat.

Sinus bradycardia is occasionally seen in normal symptomless people. The ECG is normal but the rate is slow. Sinus bradycardia is also usual in fainting attacks (vasovagal syncope). The rate in this condition is often about 40–60 beats a minute.

Vasovagal attacks are usually associated with nausea, sweating, pallor and a low blood pressure of, usually, about 60 mm Hg systolic. Most nurses who have had experience of operating theatres will, like most medical students, be familiar with the symptoms. These are the attacks that occur at the sight of blood, on prolonged standing, or in conditions of heat or exhaustion. The bradycardia is reversed by atropine and is vagal in origin. The patient should lie horizontal to maintain the circulation to the brain. Usually the patient recovers in a few minutes, but some patients will feel sick and weak for an hour or two after an attack.

HEART BLOCK

Disturbances of the conducting mechanism between the atria and ventricle are known as heart block.

First degree heart block. When the rate of conduction from the AV node down the bundle of His is prolonged, the P-R interval is longer than normal (Fig.19). This is called first degree atrio-ventricular block (AV block) or first degree heart block. This may occur temporarily in acute rheumatic fever or digitalis overdosage. In some patients it may be permanent, and is presumably due to damage to the conducting tissue by disease.

Bundle branch block is the name given to interruption of one of the main conducting bundles in the ventricles. It may affect either the left or right main bundle. It also may be permanent or temporary. When it develops in coronary thrombosis, it is evidence that the condition is affecting the conducting mechanism of the heart, and may indicate the need to take the patient to an intensive care ward and put in a pace making catheter as a precaution, in case complete block develops. The characteristic widening of the QRS complex in this condition, is due to the rapid spread of the contraction to the ventricle with an intact conducting bundle, followed by a slower spread to the other ventricle. This occurs from one cell to the next, in the same way as the impulse spreads across the normally contracting atrium. The change from a normal QRS

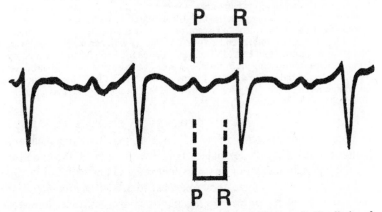

Fig.19. First degree heart block (prolongation of the P-R interval). The limits of the normal P-R interval are shown below as a box. The P-R interval on this tracing is shown above dotted down to the tracing. In this patient the cause was not known and he had no symptoms.

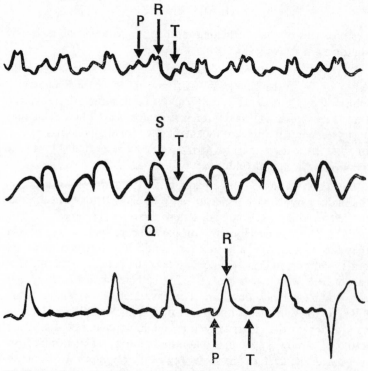

Fig.20. Bundle branch block. This shows tracings from three different patients. Tracing 1 from a man with an old coronary thrombosis. The QRS complex is represented by two R waves with a notch between them. The T wave is inverted. Tracing 2 from a patient with a recent cardiac infarct shows the QRS complex is represented by a Q wave. The S-T segment is elevated and the T wave inverted. This suggests a recent infarct and is from a patient ill with coronary thrombosis. The P wave cannot be identified. Tracing 3 the QRS complex is represented by a tall R wave followed by an inverted T wave. The P wave is easily seen but its form is variable indicating a varying sinus and nodal rhythm. This patient had no symptoms and the interruption in the conducting mechanism was probably due to a past virus infection.

complex to one showing bundle branch block (BBB) in a patient being monitored, will not make the alarm system of the monitor sound, but is an indication that the doctor should be called (Fig.20).

Incomplete heart block, sometimes called *second degree block*, is the name given to an arrhythmia in which the ventricle does not respond to every atrial beat. This may be because the atrial rate is too fast (see page 37). It may also occur when the atrial rate is normal because the AV pathway is diseased, for example by coronary artery disease, or it may be affected by drugs, especially by too much digitalis. Regular 2:1 block may occur, or the degree of dissociation may vary (Fig.21). Occasionally the AV bundle seems to get tired, the P-R interval lengthening with successive beats until

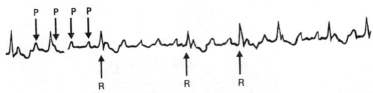

Fig.21. Varying heart block. Here the P waves are arrowed above and the QRS complex is shown by the letter R below. The pulse felt at the wrist is due to the ventricular contractions and is irregular. Although the ventricular contractions are irregular there is a constant P-R interval indicating that the ventricular beat results from atrio-ventricular conduction. The degree of block is varying. There is also first degree block.

a beat is 'dropped'—the word usually used to describe a missing ventricular beat. This is called the *Wenckebach phenomenon*. Any development of this kind in a patient being monitored needs careful watching (Fig.22).

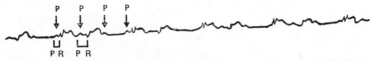

Fig.22. Wenckebach phenomenon. A tracing taken from an acutely ill patient with coronary thrombosis from which the patient died. The P waves are shown arrowed at the top and the P-R intervals below. As in figure 21 every third P wave has no following ventricular beat. The P-R interval in the first complete complex is normal, in the second the P-R interval is long, and in the third the ventricular beat is missing. The QRS complexes show bundle branch block with marked elevation of the ST segments indicating a recent infarction.

Complete heart block or complete atrio-ventricular dissociation, may be congenital or acquired, permanent or temporary. It is not uncommon as a temporary event in coronary thrombosis. When the main conducting bundle between the atria and ventricles is inter-rupted, the atria continue to beat normally, but the ventricles now beat at their own rate (Fig.23). This is commonly between 30 to 40 beats per minute. This often causes serious myocardial ischaemia

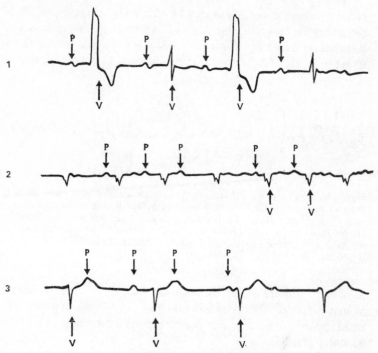

Fig.23. Complete heart block. 1. This tracing is taken from a patient with no history of coronary thrombosis. The P waves occur regularly and are not related to the QRS complexes which are shown below lettered V. Successive complexes are different, which is unusual in complete block, and indicates that the beats are starting in different parts of the ventricles. 2. A tracing from a case of cardiac infarct. There is AV dissociation and bundle branch block with Q waves. 3. Tracing of complete block probably congenital in origin.

and may need temporary or permanent pace making to increase the rate of the heart if treatment with drugs fails. In congenital heart block, however, symptoms are rare. In coronary thrombosis complete heart block usually needs emergency pace making.

CARDIAC ARREST

When the heart stops beating effectively the blood stops circulating. While an arm or leg will stand 40 minutes or more of arrested circulation, the brain will be damaged beyond recovery in a little over four minutes. It is therefore essential that a nurse can recognize the ECG patterns associated with an absent cardiac output and distinguish them from other patterns. In doing this, the first essential is to appreciate what happens when the circulation stops.

Sequence of events in cardiac arrest

The sequence of events is somewhat variable, but two features, *unconsciousness* and *progressive dilatation of the pupils* are common to all attacks. The most common sequence of events in cardiac arrest occurring spontaneously, is an inconspicuous relaxation of the patient into what could well be sleep. This occurs about 15 seconds after the arrest.The jaw may drop. Later the lips and tongue turn blue—since the circulation has stopped the oxygen gets used up. If the arrest gets this far the pupils will be beginning to dilate. Respiration stops next and by this time the patient is usually beyond help. Occasionally the arrest causes focal epileptic fits (Jacksonian epilepsy), and sometimes the patient may give a hoarse cry. When the arrest is due to an external cause such as an electric shock, there may be a fit or the patient may drop unconscious.

When the patient is connected to a monitoring ECG the machine will give an alarm when the abnormal rhythm causing the arrest begins. It is essential when the machine gives an alarm to *first look at the patient* and then at the ECG. If the patient is conscious and looking well, it is likely that the alarm is due to some fault in the connections to the machine. If however, the patient is clearly ill, the rhythm should be identified and appropriate measures taken.

Treatment of cardiac arrest

Treatment consists of measures to maintain the circulation and respiration, the identification of the nature of the onset by ECG, and appropriate treatment to restore normal rhythm.

The circulation is maintained by external cardiac massage. When this is correctly applied a pulse should be felt in the neck and groin arteries each time the chest is compressed. A normal blood pressure can be maintained by this technique for long periods.

In all cases the failure of the coronary circulation causes a rapid accumulation of lactic acid and other products of the heart metabolism in the muscle of the heart (see page 13). The resuscitation depends upon having drugs and apparatus available. Intravenous sodium bicarbonate is given, at first by injection and, as soon as possible by intravenous infusion. This physiological mild alkali is carried to the heart by external cardiac massage and counteracts the effects of acids accumulating in the heart muscle.

Respiration should be maintained initially by mouth to mouth respiration. As soon as possible, however, an endotracheal tube should be inserted by an anaesthetist, and respiration maintained with oxygen.

The combination of external cardiac massage and artificial respiration, should result in a return of the patient's colour to normal and a change in the size of the pupils of the eyes. If the pupils remain dilated or dilate further despite resuscitation, it is likely that it is too late and that, despite the heart's action, irreversible brain damage has occurred.

The ECG is recorded, preferably, by an oscilloscope. Three types of arrhythmia may be responsible for the failure of the circulation.

Causes of cardiac arrest

1. *Ventricular fibrillation* is the commonest cause of cardiac arrest (Fig.24). It may occur without warning in any heart which is

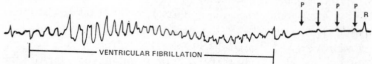

Fig.24. Ventricular fibrillation. This attack of ventricular fibrillation occurred in a woman of seventy during the recording of a routine electrocardiogram. She suffered from complete heart block and had an Adams-Stokes attack while the technician was recording the electrocardiogram. The tracing shows an initial R wave followed by an attack of ventricular fibrillation lasting about seven seconds. After this there are four P waves indicating a cessation of the ventricular fibrillation and finally the ventricle starts to beat again. This is a common type of tracing to see at the end of an attack of ventricular fibrillation. Ventricular beats return very slowly at perhaps ten or twelve a minute and gradually increase to the usual thirty to forty per minute of complete heart block.

affected by coronary thrombosis or other serious conditions. It is likely in conditions which cause serious impairment to the blood supply to the myocardium. The two most frequently encountered are, complete heart block where the bradycardia is primarily responsible, and aortic stenosis where the high ventricular pressures result in a myocardium which is more difficult to perfuse than normal. It may also be provoked by extrasystoles if the abnormal beat occurs at the time of the T wave of the preceding beat (Fig.25).

2. *Ventricular tachycardia*, if sufficiently rapid, may also cause circulatory arrest, the contractions of the ventricle occurring so

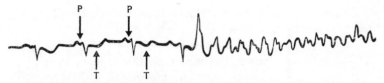

Fig.25. Cardiac arrest due to ventricular fibrillation induced by an extra systole occurring during a T wave. There are four sinus beats, the T wave in this case being inverted, and on the T wave of the fourth beat an extra systole occurs, followed immediately by four beats of ventricular tachycardia. This quickly changed to ventricular fibrillation. The tracing was recorded during cardiac catheterization on a tape recorder and subsequently played back through a direct writing machine to obtain this tracing.

rapidly that the mitral valve cannot function efficiently—the ventricle repeatedly beats when the valve is open, so that what little blood as has entered the ventricle is driven back again into the atrium by the contraction (Fig.26).

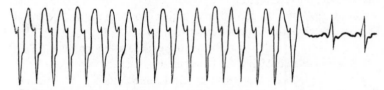

Fig.26. Ventricular tachycardia causing unconsciousness. In this attack the ventricle beat so quickly that no effective contraction occurred. The complexes are large R-S waves and the P waves due to the atrial beat can be made out here and there on the tracing. Compare this with fig.18 where the rate was slower and the patient was aware of anginal pain in the chest, but remained conscious.

3. *Asystole* is less common. The ECG shows no electrical activity. or only an occasional low voltage QS pattern (Fig.27).

All these arrhythmias *may* end spontaneously after a few seconds. The longer they last, however, the more likely they are to continue or end in irreversible arrest.

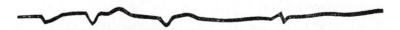

Fig.27. Asystole. The voltage remains constant about the iso-electric line, interrupted only by minute Q waves which do not represent any active ventricular contraction. This patient did not recover.

Treatment of arrhythmias. Not infrequently these arrhythmias will respond to a firm blow on the chest, or to the chest compression of cardiac massage. A conscious patient should be told to cough loudly, as this will also restore normal rhythm in many cases.

If these simple measures fail the next step depends upon the ECG. Ventricular fibrillation and ventricular tachycardia should be treated by a defibrillator, preferably of the DC type. A condenser charge of 200 to 400 joules is discharged through the chest, one electrode being placed over the right nipple area, the other in the left axilla, level with the apex of the heart. This shock will, of course, be recorded by the ECG which will be deflected off the screen. After a second or two it should return to the screen. During this time cardiac massage and respiration are maintained. If normal rhythm is not restored, the shock should be repeated. Usually the combination of maintenance of the circulation by massage, correction of myocardial acidity by bicarbonate and defibrillation is effective in ventricular fibrillation, although several shocks may be needed. In ventricular tachycardia drugs such as lignocaine, procaine amide or practolol may be needed in addition, particularly in patients in whom the arrhythmia persistently recurs.

Asystole is much more difficult to treat. In a few patients a heart beat is stimulated each time the chest is struck or compressed, and by regular blows on the chest a rhythm can be established which will continue spontaneously. However, when this technique is being tried with oscilloscope monitoring of the ECG it is essential to feel for the pulse to make sure that an effective heart beat is occurring. Quite often the blows on the chest will produce a convincing voltage change in the ECG without any corresponding mechanical contraction of the heart.

If no response occurs it is worth trying a pacemaker, initially with the external electrodes and the voltage set to 30–40 volts. If this is effective in producing a palpable pulse, it should be kept going while endocardial pacemaking is set up. All too often, however, a heart which stops with no electrical activity will not start again and resuscitation is in vain.

Stokes-Adams attacks

Transient attacks of unconsciousness of the type described are not uncommon in acquired heart block, but are very uncommon in congenital heart block which is usually a symptomless condition. They may also occur in aortic stenosis. These short attacks, lasting for a few seconds up to a minute or so, may be due to ventricular fibrillation, ventricular tachycardia, or asystole. Normal rhythm is recovered spontaneously, but the patient suffers from transient dizziness or transient unconsciousness. They are called Stokes-Adams attacks. In heart block, increasing the heart rate by Saventrine or an artificial pacemaker will usually prevent attacks, by improving the blood supply to the heart muscle (page 92). In aortic stenosis, these syncopal attacks are a warning that the condition is serious and needs urgent surgical treatment.

THE ELECTROCARDIOGRAM OF CARDIAC INFARCTION

Three changes are typical of cardiac infarction (Fig.28,29). They are the appearance of the Q wave, elevation of the S-T segment, and inversion of the T wave. These changes are seen in most patients

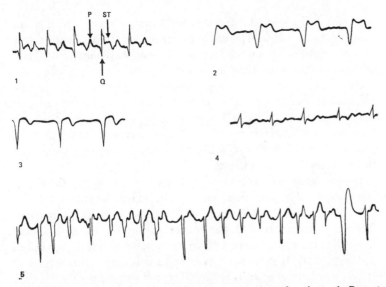

Fig.28. Acute cardiac infarct. Tracings from a number of patients. 1. Recent infarct showing a long P-R interval, Q wave, raised S-T segment and early T wave inversion. 2. Deep Q wave, widened QRS complex and elevated S-T segment. 3. The same patient as in (2) showing the same complexes a few days later. The Q wave still present, QRS interval now normal and T wave beginning to invert. 4. S-T depression with atrial fibrillation. Sinus rhythm returned spontaneously. 5. An irregular tachycardia probably nodal. Occasional P waves occur but most are lost in the ventricular complexes.

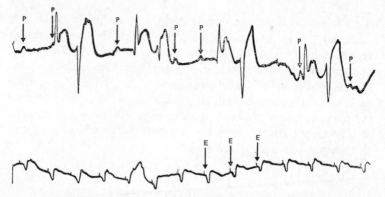

Fig.29. Heart block in an acute infarct. Bizarre ectopic beats are occurring in pairs unrelated to the P waves. In the lower tracing the rhythm after temporary pacing is shown. The impulse from the pacemaker appears as a tiny vertical stroke just before each Q wave. On the oscilloscope the pacemaker impulse appeared as a fine line flashing vertically off the screen but the stylus of the direct recorder does not move fast enough to show this. The broad fuzzy appearance of parts of these tracings is due to the movements of the patient.

who have had a cardiac infarction and there is usually a predictable progression of events. The earliest changes are the appearance of a Q wave with S-T elevation. This may be seen within an hour or two of the occurrence of chest pain and in certain patients may even precede the appearance of chest pain. As the infarct progresses, recovery is usually associated with a fall in the raised S-T segment towards normal. As the S-T segment falls, the T wave inverts, so that the final pattern is usually a Q wave followed by an inverted T wave. This is well shown in Fig.20 tracing 2, where bundle branch block complicates the picture.

It is possible to determine with considerable accuracy the site of the cardiac infarction from the leads in which the changes occur. This however, is not a concern of the nurse on a Recovery Unit. The vital matter is that the nurses caring for patients should appreciate the sort of change in an electrocardiogram that indicates serious trouble. It should also be realized that the electrocardiogram is only a voltage change. It is, therefore, not surprising that there are other causes of the changes which have just been described besides cardiac infarction. They can be due to such conditions as pulmonary embolism or virus infections affecting the heart. In addition, severe changes in the blood electrolytes can produce changes which are precisely similar to those caused by cardiac infarction. This is not surprising since the voltage changes occur as a result of alterations in the heart chemistry and this is dependent on many things besides the blood supply. In cardiac infarction the blood supply is interrupted, but in such conditions as pulmonary embolism and electrolyte imbalance, the chemistry of the heart is equally upset. We may now turn to one or two causes of an abnormal electrocardiogram which are nothing to do with the patient.

ARTEFACTS IN THE ELECTROCARDIOGRAPHIC TRACING

Most nurses who have worked on an Intensive Care Unit will be vividly familiar with electrocardiograms that do not really help, because the tracing is severely distorted by oscillations which seem to have nothing to do with the patient. It is not really possible to deal with everything that can happen here, but a few of the abnormal electrocardiograms are suitably illustrated here (Fig.30). The picture should be compared with the normal tracings and an account of

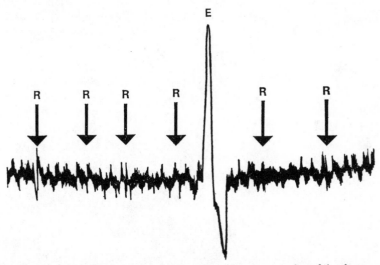

Fig.30. Artefacts on oscilloscope tracings. This oscilloscope tracing of the electrocardiogram shows alternating current interference from nearby machinery, in this case an x-ray set. The electrocardiogram is difficult to decipher because of the 50 cycle alternation but most of the QRS complexes can be made out although their form is quite obscured by the oscillations. One ventricular extra systole is easily recognizable. This sort of interference can be cured by adequate screening of the offending piece of equipment. The QRS complexes have been lettered R. The extrasystole E. The patient had atrial fibrillation.

how to deal with the situation is given later in the book on page 124. The three causes most likely to produce severe interference are the accidental detachment of a lead to the patient, the drying up of the contact between the patient's skin and the ECG electrode, and interference from nearby electrical equipment. A further common source of interference is the effect of touching the patient. Very commonly if the patient's skin is touched, for example, when a nurse is attending to him, a violent AC interference occurs. Finally, heart muscle is not the only muscle which produces a voltage change when it contracts. Any limb muscle which is active produces electrical changes and movements of the patient, and in particular shivering or tremor, such as is found in Parkinsonism, will produce oscillations on the tracing which are nothing to do with the heart. Some of these are illustrated.

6

Congenital heart disease

Congenital heart disease is a large subject and no attempt to deal with it in detail will be made here. It is an important one, however, as about 7 babies in every 1,000 are born with congenitally deformed hearts. Before embarking on this chapter the reader should read again the section on the development of the heart (page 1 to page 10). Although there is no end to the things that may be wrong with the heart in congenital heart disease, the symptoms which it causes are relatively few, and depend upon the nature of the defect in the heart. With a minor lesion there may be no symptoms in a person who lives out a normal life. At the other end of the scale, the heart may be so badly deformed that extra-uterine life is impossible, and the infant dies at birth. Between these extremes lies a range of disability, extending from heart failure in infancy, to heart failure coming on in late adult life in a patient whose childhood was apparently normal. Other patients may live a life of several decades with indifferent health throughout their life. Beginning with babies, the main symptoms are described below.

THE MAIN SYMPTOMS

Failure to thrive is the commonest symptom of serious congenital heart disease in infancy. The baby does not gain weight normally, and may never make up its birth weight. It is possible for a baby with an easily treated lesion to weigh under its birth weight at the age of 3 months.

Dyspnoea is a common and serious symptom. Many conditions cause lung congestion, with consequent breathlessness. In these infants the lungs are constantly congested by the heart disease. Attacks of heart failure are frequent and, since these increase the congestion, are frequently mistaken for 'bronchitis'. In severe cases the respiration rate may be 60–80 per minute.

Tachycardia is common in infants with severe heart disease. The rapid heart rate usually accompanies tachypnoea (rapid breathing), but may be found in infants with complicated heart disease who are so weak that they make little respiratory effort.

Sweating is common in infants with tachypnoea and tachycardia. The failure to thrive in such babies is usually due to high energy need rather than poor feeding. The sweat dissipates the heat generated by the work of the heart and of breathing.

Lung congestion is common as a symptom of left heart failure.

Liver enlargement is the common symptom of right heart failure.

Pitting oedema is unusual in babies in right heart failure. A rapid gain in weight in such children, however, suggests that oedema fluid is accumulating.

Chest deformity with a prominent pouted chest is common in severe congenital heart disease. It is due to the big heart pushing the sternum out.

Cyanosis means blue. In congenital heart disease there may be *peripheral cyanosis* due to slowing of the circulation, or *central cyanosis*, due to venous blood appearing in the systemic system as a result of the heart lesions. Both central and peripheral cyanosis may be permanent or intermittent, for example, the patient may be pink at rest and become blue on exercise, or on feeding, or when crying. It is important to look for this when babies cry or feed.

Clubbing of the fingers and toes occurs when central cyanosis is considerable. It is not solely due to cyanosis, and is also caused by chronic infections, subacute bacterial endocarditis, cancer of the lung etc. The nails become curved, and the terminal phalanges of the fingers become bulbous.

Chest pain may occur from angina in infants, or in older patients with congenital heart disease. It is difficult to detect in infants, but an observant mother or nurse may recognize chest pain if, for example, a cyanosed infant during an attack of deep cyanosis cries while drawing up its knees and pushing its hands into its chest.

In older patients the symptoms of congenital heart disease may be very difficult to establish, especially in older children. This is simply because the range of normal performance is so wide. When a child is able to run without distress and play school games well, it may be difficult to persuade the parents that the correction of a defect will result in a gain in weight and an improved athletic performance. However, it is common to find it is so.

The symptoms in congenital heart disease in older patients, range from progressive heart failure developing over months or years, to a total absence of symptoms. This range depends partly on the seriousness of the lesion and partly on the reaction of the lungs to the conditions in the heart.

DISORDERS OF CONGENITAL HEART DISEASE

The disorders of congenital heart disease may be considered in two broad groups—those in which the heart chambers are all present and correctly placed, and those in which the anatomy is disturbed, either because part of the heart has failed to form, or because the heart has developed with the connections wrongly made. It must also be appreciated that several abnormalities may be present in combination.

Hearts with a normal lay-out

In hearts which have a normal basic lay-out the abnormalities are largely (1) the presence of abnormal communications between the two sides, and (2) the presence of abnormal narrowings in the heart.

1. SEPTAL DEFECTS. If the septa which normally separate the two sides of the heart are incomplete, the natural effect is for blood to flow from the high pressure side to the low pressure side. This passage of blood from one side of the heart to the other is called a *shunt*.

In simple septal defects the shunt is from left to right. That is from the high to the low pressure side. It may occur between the atria, between the ventricles, between the first part of the aorta and pulmonary artery or through a patent ductus. They may be tabulated so:

Site of Defect	Name	Abbreviation
Atrium	Atrial septal defect	ASD
Ventricle	Ventricular septal defect	VSD
First part of aorta	Aorto-pulmonary window	—
Descending arch of aorta	Patent ductus arteriosus	PDA

In all cases the blood shunted passes through the lungs for a second time and reaches the left side of the heart again. In PDA only the lungs are traversed. In VSD the right ventricle is also over-loaded, while in ASD the right atrium and right ventricle transmit the shunted blood.

Symptoms in these conditions are very variable. The dominant complaint, as might be expected, is breathlessness. This may present as gross dyspnoea in an infant aged a few days or weeks, leading to heart failure and death in the first year of life. Other patients may lead apparently normal lives until they are 30 or 40 years old and then become dyspnoeic. Others may live a normal life span with no symptoms.

The course in any individual is determined mainly by the size of the shunt, and the reaction of the lung arteries to it. The reaction of the pulmonary arteries is not well understood. In some children the pressure in the arteries remains normal despite large shunts through the lungs. In other children, for no known reason, the shunt stimulates the arteries of the lungs to contract. This causes the pulmonary artery pressure to rise, and so the shunt to diminish. The rise in pressure is due to combination of the increased flow through the lungs and an increase in the resistance of the blood vessels, mainly the arterioles (see page 18). If the pulmonary vascular resistance (PVR) goes on rising, the shunt will diminish until no shunt occurs either way. This is called a *balanced shunt*. Further increase in the PVR will cause the shunt to reverse, so that instead of being left to right (L-R), it is now right to left (R-L). This is called a reversed shunt or *Eisenmenger reaction*. This causes central cyanosis. It is an almost absolute contra-indication to surgery, as the reversal of the shunt means that the defect is now acting as a safety valve and surgical closure of this defect will kill the patient.

The blood passing through these defects will produce characteristic noises, or *murmurs*, as they are usually called. In general the noise will be produced by blood running through from a high pressure chamber to a low pressure chamber, particularly if the hole is small. If the defect is very large or the pressure difference small, there will be little or no noise. Therefore a small VSD will make much noise. In a large VSD or if the shunt is balanced (i.e. the pressures in the right and left ventricles are equal), there may be very little noise. A loud murmur may cause a vibration which can be felt with the palm of the hand on the chest wall. This is called a *thrill*.

2. ABNORMAL NARROWINGS. Abnormal narrowings in congenital heart disease usually occur at the site of the valves.

Valve stenosis. They may affect the valve itself when the condition is called valve stenosis, or lie above it, called supravalvular stenosis, or below it, called infravalvular stenosis. The most commonly affected valves are the pulmonary and aortic valves. Stenosis requires a higher pressure to force the blood through the valve, so the muscle of the chamber proximal to the valve thickens with consequent changes in the electrocardiogram. For example, this will show left ventricular hypertrophy in aortic valve stenosis and right ventricular hypertrophy in pulmonary valve stenosis. The blood passing through the narrowing will cause a vibration like water coming through a partially turned off water tap. This will be heard as a murmur and may be enough to be felt as a thrill.

The *symptoms of valve stenosis* are few and mainly due to the reduction in heart output caused by the narrowing. In pulmonary valve stenosis, the patient may have peripheral cyanosis, because the low output causes slowing of the circulation. Other patients may get dizzy turns, particularly when standing still and working, for example while washing. In babies and children the high pressure on the right side of the heart may keep the foramen ovale open with R-L shunting through it. This causes central cyanosis. In infants with this severe stenosis, sudden death may occur.

In aortic valve stenosis, the patient is often symptomless for many years and is usually capable of violent exertion, such as playing competitive games like football. Fainting attacks may be the first symptom, indicating that the thickened left ventricle is suffering from a failure of its blood supply. Sudden death may occur, often during exertion. These symptoms may occur in childhood or be delayed until late adult life. Angina pectoris (see page 12) is another common symptom indicating that treatment is needed.

Coarctation of the aorta. This is a convenient place to mention another narrowing in the circulation which is not, strictly speaking, a deformity of the heart, although its occurrence is a consequence of the development of the heart. Coarctation of the aorta is a tight narrowing or total obstruction of the aorta at the place where the ductus arteriosus joins the last part of the aortic arch. This is usually just beyond the origin of the left subclavian artery. This obstruction to the passage of blood to the lower part of the body has to be by-passed if life is to continue. All the arteries which can form a bridge past the narrowing enlarge. The main ones are the internal mammary arteries and the upper intercostal arteries. Infants with coarctation of the aorta may sometimes develop heart failure in the first few days of life, but soon recover with treatment and develop normally. More often they are apparently normal infants.

As they get older the blood pressure in the upper part of the body rises, and may be obviously raised by the time they are three or four years old. Despite the bounding pulses in the arms, the femoral pulses are absent or difficult to feel. Between the shoulder blades, the pulsation of the dilated intercostal arteries may be felt. In some cases the ductus arteriosus remains patent and enters the aorta below the coarctation. In such children the femoral pulses may be apparently normal, but the unsaturated blood entering the aorta from the pulmonary artery results in cyanosis of the lower part of the body, most evident in the blue clubbed toe nails. This differential cyanosis, as it is called, is seen in this uncommon combination. It may also be seen in some cases of patent ductus with Eisenmenger's reaction, in which the reversed flow is sometimes all into the descending aorta.

Coarctation of the aorta is a condition with few or no symptoms in children, but in later life there is a serious risk of death from heart failure, rupture of the aorta or cerebral haemorrhage, all due to the hypertension. Surgery is therefore advised as soon as it seems the child is big enough.

Tetralogy of Fallot. Combinations of septal defects and narrowings are common. One of these, the tetralogy of Fallot, will be considered here.

In tetralogy of Fallot, the essential fault in development is a combination of a ventricular septal defect with pulmonary stenosis. The narrowing is usually a double one, there is stenosis of the valve itself and, in addition, of the muscle at the lower end of the infundibulum of the right ventricle. Blood escapes from the right ventricle into the aorta. The aorta is therefore larger than normal as it is taking a larger share of the cardiac output than normal. Because of this and the narrow pulmonary artery, the aorta comes to lie astride the ventricular septum which has the defect just below the valve. The aorta is said to 'over-ride' the septum. The right ventricle hypertrophies, as it is having to work at the same pressure as the left in order to get the blood into the aorta. These four components ventricular septal defect, pulmonary stenosis, over-riding aorta and hypertrophy of the right ventricle, constitute the tetralogy. Tetra is the Greek for four. The *symptoms of the tetralogy of Fallot* follow from the anatomy. If the pulmonary stenosis is severe, the infant is born deeply cyanosed and emergency surgery will be needed to save its life. More often the colour is normal at birth, as the pulmonary valve will pass enough blood to prevent a R-L shunt developing except, perhaps when the child is crying, feeding or straining when the child looks blue. As the child becomes more active, the amount of blood that can pass to the lungs becomes inadequate so that the cyanosis becomes more frequent, and, by the time the baby is trying to walk, it is usually cyanosed all the time. Finger clubbing develops. Many children, after exertion like running, have to squat down on their heels with their arms clasped round their shins to recover. This is called squatting and although seen in any severe type of cyanotic congenital heart disease, is most common in the tetralogy of Fallot. Some children will suddenly drop to the ground apparently for the moment unconscious. Such attacks are called *drop attacks* and are most frequently seen during exertion like walking. Another very frightening symptom is the *cyanotic attack* in which the infant or child loses consciousness, going a slate grey-blue colour and may stop breathing for some seconds, recovering only slowly. Death may occur during such attacks, which are an indication for surgical treatment.

In a few children the onset of cyanosis is delayed until they are six years old or more. In these children the pulmonary valve is often normal. The stenosis is at the infundibulum and develops progressively from infancy. In one such child, the baby was investigated by the doctor when a few months old as she had a loud murmur and was thriving poorly. A ventricular septal defect was found with a pressure of 80 mm Hg in the lower part of the right ventricle, 40 mm Hg above the infundibular narrowing and 40 mm Hg in the pulmonary artery. She had a L-R shunt. At the age of seven years she began to show cyanosis on exercise. By the age of nine she was often cyanosed but she always regained normal colour in sleep. Surgery at that age corrected the defect.

Hearts with an abnormal lay-out

Defects in which the lay-out of the heart is abnormal, are almost endless in their variety. We will consider some typical examples in three sections, remembering that combinations of defects are usual. The sections, which make a useful framework for further reading are:

1. Parts of the heart missing.

2. Errors in the arterial connections.

3. Errors of venous connections.

1. PARTS OF THE HEART MISSING. *Tricuspid atresia* is a fairly common

condition in which the tricuspid valve does not form. The right ventricle is absent or is a tiny blind sac. All cases have an atrial septal defect. Blood returns from the body to the right atrium, passes to the left atrium and all blood then passes through the mitral valve to the left ventricle, which usually has both the aorta and pulmonary artery connected to it. Cyanosis is very variable in small infants with this condition. When it is extreme the babies usually die in infancy. Some children with little cyanosis at birth may survive for some years with progressive cyanosis. Surgery can only be palliative.

The first part of the pulmonary artery may fail to form normally. When it is absent the condition is called *pulmonary atresia*. The lung blood supply may be maintained by a patent ductus arteriosus or through the bronchial arteries—the systemic blood supply to the lungs. In other children the pulmonary arteries originate in the first part of the aorta when the condition is known as *truncus arteriosus*.

2. ERRORS IN ARTERIAL CONNECTIONS. The most important and commonest fault in arterial connections is *transposition of the great arteries* (often called transposition of the great vessels). There are several varieties of this condition, but in the commonest the heart chambers are placed normally. The aorta originates in the right ventricle and the pulmonary artery in the left. If the heart is other-wise normal there would be two separate circulations, one going out of the right ventricle to the body and then back to the right atrium, the other going out of the left ventricle to the lungs and back to the left atrium again. It may help the reader to draw a simple diagram to illustrate this.

Life would clearly be impossible with this abnormality if the heart were intact. The presence of septal defects in the heart permits enough cross circulation to allow survival with very variable degrees of cyanosis, depending on the size of the defects. When these are large the cyanosis may be only slight.

3. ERRORS IN VENOUS CONNECTIONS. Errors in venous connections are quite common. Those affecting the systemic circulation are rarely important. Those affecting the lung may be very important and are essentially, the return of part or all of the blood from the lungs to the right atrium by one way or another. The usual term for this condition is *anomalous pulmonary venous drainage*. It may affect part of one lobe of a lung, a whole lobe, a whole lung, or both lungs,

when it is called *total* anomalous pulmonary venous drainage or TAPVD.

In TAPVD all the blood is returned to the right side of the heart and there must be a septal defect to allow blood to enter the left side of the heart to reach the systemic system. This is usually through an atrial septal defect. In most cases the child is only slightly cyanosed as there is an enormous volume of blood flowing through the lungs. In a typical case which was successfully treated by surgery, the lung blood flow before surgery was 17 litres a minute, the systemic flow 3·5 litres. The arterial saturation was 92 per cent instead of the normal 94–96 per cent.

TREATMENT OF CONGENITAL HEART DISEASE

Although medical treatment may assist, the most useful treatment of congenital heart disease is surgical. This may be palliative in situations where a cure is impossible or too risky, or may be a restoration of normal anatomy, which in many cases appears to be a cure. The principles underlying treatment are simple:

Defects are closed provided the Eisenmenger reaction does not make this too risky. The best results are obtained where there is a large shunt at low pressure.

Narrowings are relieved by dividing the stenosed valves or removing obstructing tissue.

Cyanosis is relieved by increasing the blood flow through the lungs by a variety of operations—pulmonary valvotomy (Brock's operation), anastomosis of the subclavian artery to the pulmonary artery (Blalock's operation), anastomosis of the aorta to the pulmonary artery (Pott's or Waterston's operation) or anastomosis of the superior vena cava to the pulmonary artery (Glenn's operation).

Pulmonary congestion in infants due to large high pressure shunts, is relieved by tying a tape round the pulmonary artery to take the pressure off the lungs. This is called *banding* the pulmonary artery.

Transposition of the great vessels is treated in infants by making an atrial septal defect. A balloon is passed through the foramen ovale into the left atrium, blown up, and then jerked sharply back into the right atrium, tearing a hole in the septum (Rashkind's operation). In suitable cases it may later be possible to create a tolerable situation by changing the venous drainage round, so that the systemic venous blood goes to the left ventricle and pulmonary venous blood to the right ventricle. The apparently easy operation of changing the great vessels back to their correct ventricles would not work, because the coronary arteries would be left being perfused by venous blood.

A comprehensive text book of congenital heart disease runs to about 900 pages. It will be evident that this chapter is only a brief summary of a few conditions. It has however, attempted to give the reader some idea of the lie of the land so that reading a text book on this subject will be made easier.

7

Rheumatic heart disease

Rheumatic heart disease is a common condition. Its cause is not fully understood, but it is related to infections with the streptococcus haemolyticus. This organism is a common cause of sore throats and tonsillitis. The typical sequence of events is a streptoccal infection, such as a sore throat, which is followed a few days or weeks later by the onset of either acute rheumatic fever or an attack of chorea.

ACUTE RHEUMATIC FEVER

Acute rheumatic fever usually begins with pain in the joints. The joints affected are mainly the ankles, knees, wrists, and elbows. Pain and tenderness comes on in one joint, lasts for a day or two and then another joint is affected, while the first joint affected often recovers. This flitting of pain from joint to joint continues. The joints suffer no permanent damage. The temperature rises, and the patient feels ill. The blood sedimentation rate rises, usually to high levels of 60 or 100 mm in one hour.

The heart is often affected by a generalized inflammation. Inflammatory cells are found throughout the muscle of the heart and the tissues of the valves. The heart rate increases and the heart enlarges. In severe cases, progressive heart failure occurs, ending in death. More usually the condition subsides after weeks or months, in many cases with complete recovery.

CHOREA

In chorea, or St Vitus's dance, the patient is afflicted with jerky uncontrollable movements affecting the whole body as a rule.

Sometimes the movements are confined to one side or mainly affect only one limb. The general symptoms are usually slight, and the heart may be only slightly affected. Repeated attacks of rheumatic fever or of chorea are not unusual.

In many patients with 'rheumatic' heart disease, no attack of acute rheumatic fever or of chorea may have occurred. In many cases, however, a sensitivity to the streptococcus or to a virus is believed to be the cause of the disease. Many people have had attacks of rheumatic fever without any effect on the heart.

EFFECTS ON THE HEART

1. Effects on the heart muscle

The effects of rheumatic heart disease are due to the inflammation in the heart. When the inflammation is severe the muscle cells are destroyed, weakening the heart muscle. In order to maintain the output of the heart with less muscle to do it, the heart dilates (Starling's law see page 16). The extent of the enlargement due to this effect may be very slight or negligible or, in other patients, may be gross. In a few patients the inflammation may slow the conduction through the atria, causing lengthening of the P-R interval. This is not uncommon in acute rheumatic fever when it is usually temporary. Occasionally it is permanent and the patient is left with permanent, usually symptomless, first degree heart block. The conducting mechanism in the ventricles is also occasionally damaged, with bundle branch block or, rarely, complete heart block resulting.

2. Effects on the valves

The effects on the valves is important, and is the result of scarring. Two main processes occur.

The edges of the valves may become stuck together by scar tissue, so that the opening becomes gradually narrowed. This progressive stenosis affects mainly the mitral and aortic valves. The tricuspid valve is less commonly affected, the pulmonary valve very rarely. The narrowing develops at a very variable rate. A few patients will progress to disabling symptoms in two or three years from an attack of rheumatic fever. More usually a patient will have had rheumatic fever in childhood, will have been found to have a cardiac murmur as a young adult, and develop symptoms fifteen or twenty years later. It is likely that gradually increasing stenosis has slowly developed over this long period.

The scarring of the valves may also produce incompetence. In the aortic valve the cusps are shortened by the scarring in their substance so that they shrink and are not big enough to meet. A similar process may reduce the size of the mitral and tricuspid valves. In these valves, however, a more important process is the shortening of the chordae tendinae which prevents the cusps meeting.

In any valve one effect may predominate so that the patient may have *pure* stenosis or *pure* incompetence of the affected valve, or, not uncommonly these processes may combine to produce a mixture of stenosis and incompetence.

The mitral valve. The valve most commonly affected is the mitral valve, and very often it is the only affected valve. The condition is more common in women than in men. The symptoms are due to the rise in left atrial pressure (LAP). At first the patient notices undue breathlessness after exercise which passes off with rest. In such a patient the LAP may be near normal at rest but will rise to 30–40 mm Hg during exercise, when the inefficient valve prevents the normal clearing of the blood pumped into the lungs by the heart.

Later the pressure in the left atrium is permanently raised with the result that the patient is short of breath at rest, and cannot lie flat (orthopnoea, see page 26). At this stage the narrowing of the valve reduces the cardiac output, the circulation slows and so more oxygen than usual is removed from the blood as it circulates through the body. In people who normally have pink dilated capillaries over the cheek bones, the slowing of the circulation causes the blood in these capillaries to become desaturated so that the blood becomes blue—a very characteristic appearance called a malar flush.

The rise in LAP is followed by a rise in pulmonary artery pressure, and eventually right heart failure. The right ventricle dilates, the tricuspid valve becomes incompetent, and the patient develops right heart failure with oedema, engorged and pulsating neck veins, and liver pulsation (see chapter 4). The slow circulation through the gut impairs digestion and the absorption of gas from the gut is impaired by the high venous pressure. Often matters are made worse by a rapid heart rate, usually due to atrial fibrillation (see page 37). The history of disability in mitral valve disease is usually one of gradually increasing breathlessness spread over many years and often attributed by the patient to 'getting older'.

The aortic valve. In contrast, aortic valve disease is often symptomless for many years. In aortic stenosis the ventricle has to work at a higher pressure than normal. In aortic incompetence the leak back in diastole causes an increase in the stroke volume, the quantity of blood being ejected at each beat being larger than normal. In combined aortic stenosis and incompetence, the ventricle has to eject a larger quantity of blood at a pressure higher than normal. The ventricle has a large reserve and tolerates this state of affairs for many years. It is commonplace to find patients with no symptoms, little change in heart size, but gross changes in the ECG. Apart from the cardiac murmurs there may be little evidence of serious disease, although the volume of the arterial pulse may provide a clue. In aortic stenosis it is usually difficult to feel, rising and falling slowly. In aortic incompetence, it is exaggerated with a wide pulse pressure. In combined aortic stenosis and incompetence, it is usually dicrotic with a double peak which may be palpable.

The symptoms which are so late in appearing are all indications for urgent treatment, as sudden death is all too common in this disease. Angina, syncopal attacks and progressive dyspnoea are common.

Combined aortic and mitral valve disease is common, the symptoms depending on which valve is the more seriously affected. Most commonly the effects on the inefficient left heart are felt by the lung, with dyspnoea and right heart failure as the dominant symptoms.

TREATMENT

Treatment is of two kinds—the treatment of heart failure (page 30) and the treatment of the valve disorders. The stenosed mitral valve is treated by parting the stuck edges with a dilator, an operation usually done 'closed', i.e. without using the heart lung machine. An incompetent or heavily calcified mitral valve is replaced. Diseased aortic valves are usually replaced. All replacements entail opening the heart or aorta, so a by-pass operation using a heart lung machine is needed.

Nursing patients with rheumatic heart disease requires a fair knowledge of the disordered heart function. It is important to remember that many patients with mitral valve disease, and some with aortic valve disease, will drown if they are nursed flat or head down. It is particularly important to remember this when patients with rheumatic heart disease have operations which are nothing to do with the heart. If after an emergency laparotomy or similar operation, a patient with rheumatic heart disease develops hypo-tension, the usual treatment of raising the foot of the bed to increase the blood pressure may cause fatal pulmonary oedema. The blood pressure must be increased by other means—transfusion or by drugs.

EMBOLISM

Embolism may occur in patients with rheumatic heart disease. This word is used to describe the blocking of an artery or arteriole, by something which has flowed along the arterial tree until the vessels become too small for it to get further. Most commonly the embolism is due to a piece of clot which forms in the left atrium in mitral stenosis, particularly if the atrium is not contracting as in atrial fibrillation. Occasionally the embolus is a fragment of calcium from the mitral or aortic valves, where these have calcified. The particle may end up in the brain, a limb artery, any visceral artery or in a coronary artery. The results depend on the artery concerned. In the brain there may be a transient paralysis, or a permanent serious stroke depending on the size of the embolus. A massive piece of clot may plug the bifurcation of the aorta and early emergency surgery is needed if the lower limbs are to be saved.

The *symptoms* in an *embolus to a limb* are sudden pain in the affected part with loss of the arterial pulse and pallor or a greyish cyanosis. Paralysis usually follows quickly if the blocked artery is a large one. Slight oedema is common. When there is a good collateral circulation round the blocked artery the limb may recover without surgery. For example, the arterial circulation round the elbow and knee is usually good enough to keep the hand or foot going, if the bifurcation of the brachial or femoral artery is blocked. In nursing, however, it is important to remember that the arteries that encircle the joints are small with low pressure in them. The affected part should not be raised above heart level if slight oedema occurs, as this may endanger the arterial supply. This contrasts with nursing a venous block in a limb, where oedema is considerable because of the normal arterial pressure. Here there is no danger to the arterial supply and elevation of the limb above the heart is beneficial.

8

Bacterial endocarditis

Bacterial endocarditis is the name given to an infection affecting the valves and lining of the heart. The infection is rare in a normal heart, and is due to bacteria present in the blood stream settling on some abnormal area of the heart, usually a diseased valve or septal defect. It is most common on the mitral and aortic valves, rare on the pulmonary valve, and very uncommon on the tricuspid valve. Patent ductus and ventricular septal defects may become infected, but atrial septal defect only very rarely. Infection is not uncommon at the site of coarctation of the aorta.

INFECTION DURING SEPTICAEMIA

The bacteria may get into the blood stream as a *septicaemia*, for example from a boil or carbuncle, or as an early stage in diseases like pneumonia or meningitis. In such cases the heart infection may be only part of a serious generalized infection. Certain bacteria, such as the staphylococcus aureus and pneumococcus, are particularly liable to settle in diseased hearts. They cause rapid destruction of the valves with disastrous consequences, rapid and severe heart failure resulting. The disease of the heart in these cases is called *acute bacterial endocarditis*.

INFECTION DURING BACTERAEMIA

More commonly the infection of the heart occurs during a *bacteraemia*. This is a symptomless blood stream infection. The most common source of the bacteria is the teeth. The bacteraemia may follow dental extractions or may occur during chewing if the tooth sockets or gums are infected. The most common infecting organism is the streptococcus viridans. For this reason all patients with congenital or rheumatic heart disease are advised to have antibiotics when they have dental treatment and are told to visit their dentist regularly.

Symptoms

The symptoms of infection with the streptococcus viridans are much less acute, and the condition is called *subacute bacterial endocarditis*. Often the first symptoms are lassitude and weakness due to the anaemia which the infection causes by depressing the formation of red blood cells. The infection will usually have been present for weeks or months before this is noticed. Other symptoms are due to small infected particles breaking away and passing to the capillaries before lodging when the blood vessel becomes too small for them to get any further. These are called emboli. They commonly cause small red spots in the skin (petechiae) or streaks beneath the finger or toe nails (splinter haemorrhages), fading after a few days. In the pulp of the fingers they may cause painful mulberry coloured lumps called Osler's nodes. Emboli in the kidney cause haematuria. The spleen enlarges, and occasionally mild finger clubbing occurs. When large particles break off, they may block a large artery in the brain or in a limb, with serious damage to function. Such large emboli may become the focus for a local abscess with the formation of an aneurysm or blow-out of the artery concerned. Because such aneurysms were wrongly thought to be due to infection with a fungus they are called *mycotic aneurysms*.

Damage to the heart valves may be slight or so serious as to be catastrophic. The usual causes of serious valve disorders are the perforation of an aortic valve cusp, leading to acute left heart failure, and rupture of the chordae tendinae causing sudden gross mitral incompetence. In both cases the patient rapidly becomes grossly dyspnoeic and acute pulmonary oedema develops, with the production of frothy, often blood stained, sputum.

TREATMENT

Treatment is directed to treating the infection and its effects. It is important to identify the infecting organism so that the correct antibiotic can be given. Repeated blood cultures may be needed before this is achieved. Antibiotic treatment is continued for 6–8 weeks, often by continuous intravenous infusion. Valve rupture may necessitate emergency surgery to replace the ruptured valve. Mycotic aneurysms usually require surgery, which may be in itself dangerous. If a limb embolism causes gangrene, amputation may be needed.

9

Coronary artery disease

There are two important components in coronary artery disease, atheroma and thrombosis.

ATHEROMA

Atheroma is a word applied to narrowing inside arteries due to small patches of fatty material which accumulate between the inner lining, the intima, and the middle layer, the media. These patches of fatty material occur in everybody as they get older, being more common in people with high blood pressure and in people who tend to develop high blood fat levels after eating foods containing fat. The atheroma patches narrow the lumen of the arteries. They are usually called atheromatous plaques.

THROMBOSIS

Thrombosis simply means clotting. Clots tend to form at the site of atheromatous plaques, where the turbulence they cause in the blood flow favours the deposition of platelets and fibrin. Clotting occurs more easily than normal when the blood is loaded with fat after a meal. For example, a breakfast of two complete rashers of bacon, a fried egg and two slices of toast with butter, will produce marked shortening of the clotting time. The effect is not uniform, as some people develop a much higher lipaemia (blood fat level) than others. Immobility and smoking cigarettes also increase the risk of thrombosis.

Angina

Both atheroma and thrombosis may cause angina when they affect the coronary arteries. Atheroma causes *angina of effort*. The patient finds that if he exerts himself faster than a certain limit, pain is produced (see page 12), as part of the heart has outrun its blood supply. If he stops or goes more slowly the pain is quickly relieved as the affected muscle recovers. The pain usually comes on more easily if the circulation is already loaded, for example in cold weather or by digestion after a meal. Coronary thrombosis usually causes *angina of infarction*. Here the pain is more severe and long lasting, and comes from the muscle whose blood supply is cut off by the clot in the coronary artery. It often comes on when the patient is at rest, and may be severe enough to make the patient sweat. In both cases the pain is usually felt as a crushing sensation inside the chest. It often radiates to the arms and may be felt down the inside of the arms to the wrists. It may also be felt in the throat or jaw. Sometimes a coronary thrombosis may occur without pain.

EFFECTS OF CORONARY THROMBOSIS

The effects of a coronary thrombosis depend upon its site and the size of the artery affected.

Myocardial infarction and its effects

Any thrombosis in a coronary artery causes myocardial infarction (death of heart muscle). Even a small infarct may cause ventricular fibrillation or asystolic arrest with death, unless external cardiac massage is given.

1. *Heart failure.* A considerable infarct will cause heart failure which may be mainly left heart failure, or right heart failure, depending upon which ventricle is mainly supplied by the artery concerned.

2. *Valve incompetence.* The dilatation of the heart resulting from the weakening of the muscle may cause mitral or tricuspid valve incompetence. Valve incompetence may also occur as a result of ischaemic damage to the papillary muscles

3. *Heart block.* The impairment of the blood supply to the heart in cardiac infarction not infrequently involves the conducting system. Bundle branch block may occur, or, less commonly, involvement of the main conducting system may cause complete heart block. The poor blood supply to the heart muscle which follows on the slow heart rate in complete block requires emergency pacing to increase the heart rate to restore the myocardial blood supply.

4. *Arrhythmias.* Similarly rapid arrhythmias may occur—atrial fibrillation, ventricular tachycardia etc. Here the blood supply to the heart muscle is also impaired—this time by the low output associated with excessive tachycardia. Emergency treatment to slow the heart is needed.

5. *Aneurysms.* Occasionally an area of the left ventricle is so thinned by the infarct that it cannot withstand the pressure in the ventricle and blows out like a balloon into a localized aneurysm of the heart wall. If this is large it greatly weakens the action of the heart, as the force of each systole is expended in blowing up the aneurysm. This causes what is called paradoxical pulsation—the cardiac aneurysm expands as the rest of the heart contracts. On rare occasions the heart wall ruptures, causing death by bleeding into the pericardial sac (tamponade).

6. *Embolisms.* A further hazard is the formation of clot on the lining of the heart where the inflammatory changes due to the natural response to death of tissue occur. Parts of this clot may break off and cause embolism, affecting the limbs or viscera or brain, if the area affected is in the left ventricle.

The heart has a natural tendency to form new blood vessels when the muscle is ischaemic, so in many patients the angina improves as blood finds its way to the ischaemic area by blood vessels coming in from neighbouring areas. In the same way, a cardiac infarct is followed by revascularization to a greater or lesser extent of the infarcted area. Considerable natural recovery is therefore usual in both angina of effort and following infarction. It must be remembered, however, that atheroma is a general conditon and usually many blood vessels are affected by this condition. Treatment, therefore, should be directed to the immediate symptoms which have brought the patient to the doctor and also, as far as possible, to the more general problem of reducing the chances of the blood clotting, and arresting the progress of the atheromatous process.

TREATMENT

The treatment may be considered under the following headings:
Immediate treatment.

1. The relief of pain.
2. Avoiding thrombosis.

3. Improving the blood supply to the heart muscle.

After care.

4. Reducing the tendency to the formation of atheroma.

5. Prevention of further infarcts.

1. Relief of pain

In *cardiac infarct*, pain is relieved by the injection of analgesics such as Morphine, Dextromoramide (Palfium) or Methadone (Physeptone).

In *angina of effort*, the simplest measure is to reduce the rate of activity and so sparing the heart. Drugs which dilate the blood vessels in the heart will also relieve angina. These are mainly nitrites. Amyl Nitrite is inhaled, Tab. Trinitrini are chewed and placed under the tongue so that the drug is absorbed from the mucous membrane of the mouth. Many proprietary preparations are based upon this drug. The main disadvantages of this treatment are the headache and dizziness which may result from generalized vasodilatation.

2. Avoiding thrombosis

In cardiac infarction the patient is at risk from:

a. Spread of the infarct in the heart.

b. Clot forming on the lining of the heart where the endocardium is involved.

c. Clots forming in the veins, mainly in the lower limbs, from immobility.

a. Spread of the infarct in the heart is probably little affected by current treatment. Anticoagulants have been given for 25 years in acute infarction, and the evidence suggests that they do little to reduce the effects of the coronary thrombosis.

b. Clots forming on the lining of the heart are lessened by anticoagulant therapy. The risk is greatest during the period of time from 3rd to 10th days after the infarction. Heparin by intravenous injection, followed by anticoagulants such as Warfarin or Sinthrone by mouth, are given. The dose is judged by measuring the prothrombin time. This is a simple laboratory test of the clotting time which measures the blood level of prothrombin, a factor in blood clot formation which is reduced by the anticoagulant.

c. Clots forming in veins are reduced by anticoagulants, by leg exercises during the day, and by early ambulation of the patient.

Thirty years ago it was usual to treat every patient by strict bed rest for three to six weeks. In many wards all patients were nursed flat, and not allowed to feed themselves for at least a week. Half the patients treated in this way died of embolism from a clot in the heart or veins. With modern treatment this is now a rare event.

3. Improving the blood supply to the heart muscle

In acute infarction this is achieved by maintaining the blood pressure after the infarct by suitable drugs and controlling the heart rate by slowing tachycardia, and increasing the rate by artificial pacing, when the rate is slowed by heart block. Slow sinus rhythm is usually due to vagal overaction (the vagus is in the 10th nerve and slows the heart). It will usually respond to injected Atropine.

Acute arrhythmias such as ventricular tachycardia, ventricular fibrillation or asystole require appropriate emergency treatment.

4. Reducing the tendency to atheroma formation

Reducing the tendency to atheroma formation is an obvious aim of after care. We do not yet know enough of the causes of atheroma to be sure of the value of treatment to prevent it. Avoidance of animal fats in the diet and the reduction of blood fat by such drugs as Clofibrate appear to be of value.

5. Prevention of further infarcts

Prevention of further infarcts is encouraged by keeping the patient active, giving long term anticoagulants, stopping cigarette smoking (20 cigarettes a day increases infarction three times), and advising the patient to avoid occupations or pastimes likely to cause stress or raise the blood pressure. Here the patient's temperature is of great importance. For example, golf is an excellent game for a man who likes a leisurely game and who does not worry about the result. It would be bad for a man who desires fiercely to win and plays every stroke as if his life depended on it. Heavy work in hot surroundings should be changed for lighter work, and an office job which ties the patient to a chair all day should, if possible, be arranged to include intermittent exercise throughout the day—going into the works to supervise or dictating letters while walking in the office. Finally, the blood pressure, if raised as a result of hypertension, should be suitably treated to bring it down.

10

Hypertensive heart disease

The pressure at which the blood circulates in the arteries, is a result of many different factors. The main ones are the cardiac output and the peripheral resistance. These two determine the pressure, but are themselves dependent on many other factors. Thus, we have seen how the change in position from lying to standing involves complicated adjustments to maintain the pressure in the arteries supplying the brain (see page 21). This adjustment of the state of vasoconstriction or vascular tone is under many different controls, which are both chemical and nervous. For example, the blood pressure and heart rate rise when people are nervous. If patients in bed in a ward are connected to recording apparatus, it is found that as the doctors do a ward round the blood pressure goes up as they approach any patient's bed and falls again as they move on past it. It follows that a measurement of blood pressure may give a low reading on one occasion and a high one on another, both being 'normal' for the circumstances in which it was taken.

This variability in blood pressure makes the definition of the 'normal' pressure difficult. The usual figure quoted for systolic pressure is 120 mm Hg (millimetres of mercury) and for diastolic pressure 80 mm Hg. This is about 2 pounds per square inch. Most insurance companies accept a pressure of 140/95 mm Hg as normal in someone being examined for the first time by a stranger. Many people have lower pressures than this, 100/70 mm Hg being the usual limit, although occasional healthy people have systolic pressures below 100 mm Hg.

HYPERTENSION

A sustained high blood pressure is called hypertension. It is due to an increase in the tone of the arterioles, the cardiac output being normal.

The diastolic pressure is the best measure of the condition, since a high systolic pressure can occur in anyone as the aorta gets less elastic with age. The continually increased arteriole tone results in hypertrophy of the wall of the arterioles, which become thicker than normal.

Causes

The causes of hypertension are many. Acute or chronic kidney disease may cause high blood pressure. A few cases are due to tumours of the suprarenal tissue which secrete adrenalin and noradrenalin. These are called phaeochromocytomas. Increased secretion may also occur in Cushing's syndrome. Coarctation of the aorta is an uncommon cause. In most cases there is no obvious cause and in these patients the condition is called 'benign' *essential hypertension.*

Effects

1. *Atheroma formation.* Continued hypertension results in an increased formation of atheroma with narrowing of the lumen of the arteries, weakening of the arterial walls especially in the aorta which enlarges, and lengthening of the arteries which therefore tend to become tortuous. Weakened arteries may rupture, especially in the brain, causing strokes, and the atheroma results in a greater risk of thrombosis than in a normotensive person (one with a normal blood pressure) of the same age. The arterial damage in the kidney may provoke changes causing the kidney to become ischaemic and so raise the pressure higher by increasing its secretion of renin. Progressive kidney damage may also end in failure of the kidney with uraemia.

2. *Acute necrosis.* Not infrequently the pressure causes acute necrosis in the arterioles and this results in a rapidly rising hypertension with progressive renal failure. In these patients papilloedema (swelling of the optic disc) occurs. When this series of changes is present the patient is said to have *malignant hypertension.*

3. *Hypertrophy of left ventricle wall.* The first effect of hypertension on the heart is thickening or *hypertrophy* of the wall of the left ventricle. This is a natural result of constantly maintaining a pressure higher than normal. In many patients this is quite symptomless and many people have hypertension for years without symptoms. Some may complain of headaches, usually worse in the morning, and

usually felt in the front of the head. The heart may be a little enlarged and the electrocardiogram may show left ventricular hypertrophy with, sooner or later, a strain pattern—depression of the S-T segments with T wave inversion in leads 1, AVL and the V leads in the left axilla.

4. *Dyspnoea.* The continued load on the ventricle eventually leads to failure of the left ventricle with a rise in left atrial pressure and consequent breathlessness. In this stage the patient may find that exertion causes acute shortness of breath, so that they have to stop, gasping to get their breath back. At a later stage this breathlessness occurs at night when lying down and they have to sit on the edge of the bed to recover. This dyspnoea is very distressing and is sometimes called cardiac asthma. The attacks of dyspnoea at night are called paroxysmal nocturnal dyspnoea. The changes in the lung causing the dyspnoea, are the same as those operating in the lung in mitral valve disease and aortic valve disease, and are directly due to the rise in left atrial pressure. Mitral valve incompetence may result from dilatation of the left ventricle.

5. *Failure of right heart.* If the hypertension continues, the rise in left atrial pressure is followed by a rise in the pulmonary artery pressure and eventual failure of the right side of the heart with raised jugular venous pressure, liver enlargement, oedema, and renal congestion and failure. The sequence of events has been described earlier (see page 28).

At any stage the sequence of events may be interrupted by a sudden catastrophe due to the effects of the raised blood pressure on the arteries. For example, the hypertension may cause cerebral haemorrhage, or renal failure. The aorta may form an aneurysm which may rupture. The atheroma in the coronary arteries may result in coronary thrombosis.

Investigation

Investigation is directed first to identifying possible treatable causes. Coarctation can usually be diagnosed on examination by the absence of pulses in the femoral arteries, and the presence of palpable collateral arteries between the shoulder blades. The kidney function is investigated first by testing for albumen and examining the deposit for casts and cells. If these are present it is necessary to decide whether they are the result of renal disease, which is causing hypertension, or hypertension causing renal disease. It may be necessary to examine the kidney by taking a biopsy or get pictures of the renal tract by intravenous pyelogram. In this investigation an injection of x-ray contrast medium is given. This is excreted by the kidneys and x-ray pictures show the pelvis of the kidney, the ureters and the bladder. X-ray pictures of the arteries to the kidneys may be obtained by injection of contrast medium through a catheter passed up the aorta to the renal arteries, from a puncture of the femoral artery.

Cushing's syndrome is usually easily recognized by the patient's characteristic appearance, but in this condition and in phaeochromocytoma, measurements of the catecholamines excreted in the urine may be made.

A diagnosis of benign essential hypertension is usually reached by exclusion of other known causes.

TREATMENT

The treatment of hypertension depends upon the cause. Where a cause can be identified this is treated. Coarctation can be resected, phaeochromocytoma removed, and renal disease, in a few cases where this is possible, treated.

In many cases treatment is directed to relieving anxiety by barbiturate or tranquillizers, and in patients in whom this is the main cause of raised blood pressure, the treatment is very effective.

In most cases the cause of the hypertension is not understood, and treatment is directed to lowering the blood pressure by drugs. Many of these work by reversing the high arteriolar tone which maintains the patient's raised blood pressure. This affects the patient's ability to compensate for changes in position, so that the blood pressure is lower when they stand up. In such treatment the blood pressure must be measured with the patient standing up as well as lying down, as too much of the drug will cause the blood pressure to fall so low when they stand, that dizziness occurs when they are in this position.

Effective treatment can reverse malignant hypertension in patients who react well to the treatment. Lives are prolonged, and many people can continue useful working lives for years, in a condition in which progressive disability and heart failure or sudden catastrophe used to occur in the days before such treatment became available.

11

Myocarditis, cardiomyopathy, cor pulmonale, syphilis, and pulmonary embolism

In this chapter a number of unrelated conditions may be dealt with briefly. Most of them are not well understood and the first two, myocarditis and cardiomyopathy, are not single diseases, but groups of diseases which resemble each other.

MYOCARDITIS

Myocarditis simply means inflammation of the heart muscle. The muscle of the heart is affected by an inflammatory process, with patches of inflammatory cells in the heart muscle and disruption of the muscle cells. The heart is weakened and therefore enlarges. The common causes are probably mostly virus infections of many different kinds—for example, acute heart failure killed many people in the great epidemic of Asian influenza. Acute heart failure, occasionally with atrial fibrillation may be seen in the toxaemia of pneumonia, especially when due to severe infections with the pneumococcus or Friedländer's bacillus.

Recovery usually depends upon the damage to the muscle in the acute stage. Most patients recover to continue with a normal life span, the heart may be remaining permanently a little larger than it was before the illness. Atrial fibrillation or ventricular conduction defects, such as bundle branch block or complete heart block, may persist permanently. In a few patients a gradual progression to irreversible heart failure occurs, either because of progressive damage to the heart, or because the initial damage to the muscle exceeded the reserve of the myocardium.

CARDIOMYOPATHY

Cardiopathy means 'heart muscle disease', and is applied to a number of obscure disorders. Chief among them is one termed *hypertrophic obstructive cardiomyopathy*. This strange complaint is most commonly seen in the left ventricle, much less often in the right. The normal co-ordination of muscle contraction which ejects the blood from the ventricle into the aorta is disturbed, so that the muscle below the aortic valve contracts too early in the systole of the ventricle. This contraction at the outflow of the ventricle obstructs the ejection of blood, causing the muscle of the body of the ventricle to hypertrophy. This induces hypertrophy in the obstructing muscle, so that the walls of the whole chamber become thicker and thicker. Sudden death may occur. In early cases the abnormal contraction can be prevented by giving drugs that stop the action of nerve cells (the beta type of adrenergic cells). These patients are therefore treated by beta blocking agents such as Practolol.

The term cardiomyopathy is applied to a number of other rare conditions.

COR PULMONALE

Cor pulmonale means 'the heart due to lung disease'. In any chronic lung disease in which there is progressive impairment of the lung capacity to oxygenate blood, the heart will suffer from the inadequate supply of oxygenated blood. The lung disability may be either a great reduction in the area of lung available for oxygenation, or a failure of the air breathed to reach all parts of the lung, or a mixture of these effects. In the first case where lung tissue has been destroyed by, for example, cystic disease, pulmonary tuberculosis, or emphysema, the patient oxygenates the blood normally in the remaining lung, but the loss of lung oxygenating area means that the blood has to pass through a smaller system than normal. The pressure in the lung arteries rises, and the right side of the heart may fail.

When the air fails to reach all parts of the lung evenly, some blood will pass through lung where there is not enough oxygen. This blood will not be normally oxygenated and will reach the left side of the heart still desaturated. The patient will therefore be cyanosed. This cyanosis will be a central cyanosis as the blood is leaving the heart incompletely oxygenated (see page 27). Impaired distribution of air in the lung may be due to bronchial obstruction, bronchial asthma, bronchopneumonia or, once more, emphysema. The reaction of the body to the inadequate arterial oxygen supply in this condition is similar to that seen in anaemia—the output of the heart increases and the formation of more red blood cells is stimulated. In this condition the patient therefore develops polycythaemia (many blood cells) and a high cardiac output. Polycythaemic blood in which the haemoglobin may be 130–140 per cent and the haematocrit (the packed cell volume) nearly double normal, is much more viscid than normal. The combination of having to maintain a higher than normal output with inadequate oxygen supply to the myocardium, and having to pump round blood which is far more sticky than normal, also causes heart failure.

Treatment is primarily a matter of trying to improve lung function. Curable diseases are few. Oxygen will help most patients—but in a few who are habituated to abnormal blood gas tensions, the administration of oxygen causes them to stop breathing adequately and carbon dioxide may have to be given with the oxygen. General measures for treating heart failure—diuretics etc. are also used. Where a treatable cause like asthma is present, enormous improvement is possible with a great reduction in heart size as the patient's condition improves.

One very important warning. Cor pulmonale is a distressing condition. Many drugs used to treat distress such as barbiturates and morphine, depress respiration. They should be given with great caution to patients in heart failure from cor pulmonale.

SYPHILIS

Syphilis was the name of a shepherd boy in a story. It is now applied to the disease he was supposed to have had. It is caused by a spirochaete, the treponema pallidum. It very rarely affects the heart directly. Syphilis causes two important changes in the aorta. One is disorganization and destruction of the wall so that the aorta dilates. The dilatation may be general in character, causing what is called a *fusiform aneurysm*, or part of the wall may give way, blowing up like a balloon on the side of the aorta. This is called a *saccular aneurysm*. These aneurysms may cause pain by eroding the vertebrae or sternum. If the dilatation involves the aortic valve ring, the valve will leak. Finally, the aneurysm may burst, or rupture, to use the more usual medical word.

The second effect of syphilis on the aorta is an increase in the thickness of the lining or intima. This may get so thick that the branches of the aorta are blocked at their origin. This may cause angina if it involves the coronary arteries, or trouble in the upper limbs or the brain if the branches to these structures are involved.

Treatment for syphilis is by Penicillin, Arsenic, Bismuth, and Mercury preparations. These may have to be given cautiously if the patient has angina, since they can cause swelling of the syphilitic tissues. This could have disastrous results in someone with partial obstruction to the coronary arteries. This swelling is called a Herxheimer reaction. Saccular aneurysms may be removed and fusiform ones plicated surgically.

PULMONARY EMBOLISM

The problem of embolism in heart disease has been mentioned on page 69. Pulmonary embolism is an important cause of ill health and death. The usual course of events is the formation of a clot in a systemic vein, for example in the leg or pelvis. The clot grows into a ribbon like accumulation of platelets, red cells and fibrin attached to the place where it began. At this stage it is like a piece of ribbon sea weed being washed by the tide. Sooner or later it breaks off and is carried in the circulation through the heart into the lungs where it blocks up the artery. The common causes of this type of clot formation are *immobility*, as in the treatment by absolute bed rest, *local infection*, as in appendicitis, or *pelvic masses*, as in pregnancy. In the days when patients with cardiac infarction were nursed by absolute bed rest for six weeks, half the deaths were due to embolism. Similarly in the days when patients were kept strictly in bed for ten days after having their appendix out, embolism killed far more people than did the operation or the appendicitis. The main reason for the reduction in the number of deaths from embolism are early ambulation of the patients and making all patients confined to bed do regular leg exercises to keep the blood moving.

There are two main types of pulmonary embolism.

1. *Massive pulmonary embolism.* In the first, usually called massive pulmonary embolism, the clot forms a tangled mass which blocks off one or both main pulmonary arteries. The patient may die in a few minutes, or if the block is not complete, become suddenly desperately ill and cyanosed. The electrocardiogram shows acute changes, The extent of the block may be shown by angiocardiography and the clot removed by emergency surgery. Investigation and surgery have usually to be done within an hour or two of the episode if the life is to be saved.

2. *Multiple pulmonary emboli.* The second type of illness occurs when the clot breaks off as it forms so that many small emboli occur. These are called multiple pulmonary emboli. The patient becomes increasingly short of breath with progressively increasing pressure in the pulmonary artery. Cyanosis is usually a late symptom and death is usually due to right heart failure.

12

Diseases of the pericardium

The pericardium is the name given to the membranes which cover the heart. It is a double layer forming a closed sac. The layer which covers the heart is called the epicardium and consists of a glistening smooth surface of epithelium attached to the heart by connective tissue. Around the veins and arteries entering the heart this membrane is turned back over itself and the smooth epithelial surface is continued to cover the heart with a second layer called the pericardium. The movements of the beating heart are made easier by this double layer, which is lubricated by serous fluid just like the pleura and the peritoneum. The space between the layers of pericardium is called the pericardial sac and corresponds to the pleural cavity of the lung covering and the abdominal cavity of the peritoneum. As with the pleura and peritoneum, the epicardium is often called the visceral layer of the pericardium and the outer layer called the parietal layer. There are no pain nerve endings in the visceral layer, but the parietal layer has pain nerve endings so that acute infections affecting this layer cause pain. Infections of the parietal pleura cause the pain of 'pleurisy' and infections of the parietal pericardium cause the pain of 'pericarditis'.

The pericardium envelops the heart and is slack enough to permit the normal changes in heart size. When the heart enlarges slowly as a result of disease the pericardium stretches to allow this. It will, however, prevent rapid enlargement. If fluid accumulates rapidly in the pericardial space, for example, an inflammatory exudate in pericarditis, or blood in trauma, or rupture of the heart, the fluid in the pericardium prevents the filling of the heart This is known as *tamponade*.

ACUTE PERICARDITIS

Acute pericarditis is usually due to infection. The commonest form seen is *acute benign pericarditis*, which is probably a virus infection. The patient presents with acute pain in the chest, which may radiate to the shoulder tip. The electrocardiogram shows changes which may resemble those of acute cardiac infarction. The effusion is usually small and a pericardial friction rub, due to the roughened pericardial surfaces grating against each other as the heart beats, is common. The condition usually responds rapidly to treatment with steroids, but may relapse, and recurrences are not uncommon for as long as a year or eighteen months after the initial attack. The fluid is a sterile yellow, clear or slightly cloudy, with a high protein content in which a clot forms as it cools after removal. A similar pericardial effusion is common in acute rheumatic fever.

Infective pericarditis may also occur if a pleurisy or pneumonia occurs adjacent to the heart. In these cases the fluid may be infected or sterile. On rare occasions, pus is found and usually needs to be drained surgically, like an empyema in the pleural cavity.

Pericarditis with a thick layer of fibrin on the pericardium may occur in severe uraemia. There is usually a loud friction rub, which may be palpable to the palm of the hand placed on the chest wall over the heart. It differs from the usual thrill caused by a loud murmur, in that it is felt throughout the cardiac cycle.

As has been mentioned tamponade may occur if any large effusion accumulates rapidly in the pericardium. This prevents the adequate filling of the heart and so reduces the cardiac output. The signs are a rising filling pressure, evident from the rising level of the venous pressure in the neck veins, an increasing heart rate and, eventually, a falling arterial pressure. Urgent aspiration of fluid from the pericardial sac is needed to treat this condition.

A slowly accumulating pericardial effusion may cause great dilatation of the pericardial sac without tamponade. This condition is uncommon and its cause unknown. The very large shadow of the heart on x-ray in this condition, often raises the possibility that the patient is suffering from congenital heart disease. It is treated surgically by removing the parietal layer of the pericardium.

CONSTRICTIVE PERICARDITIS

If a chronic fibrosing process affects the pericardium, it reduces the extent to which the heart can fill and so reduces its output. This results in chronic heart failure. The patient usually has signs of severe right sided heart failure with engorged neck veins and an enlarged liver. Oedema of the ankles is often slight. Evidence of left heart failure is uncommon. When it occurs it is due to a reduction of the cardiac output, the patient complaining of dizzy turns or fainting. Evidence of pulmonary venous hypertension is almost unknown and the patients can usually sleep flat without distress. This is because the constriction reduces the blood entering the right side of the heart. The left heart has usually little difficulty in passing on what blood reaches it. Atrial fibrillation occurs in about 25 per cent of patients.

The commonest cause of constrictive pericarditis is tuberculosis. In an acute tuberculous infection, any of the serous cavities may be involved, and arthritis, peritonitis, pleurisy or pericarditis with effusion may occur. Recovery from tuberculous pericarditis is followed by severe scarring and contraction, constricting the pericardium. Marked calcification may occur, making the diagnosis easy as the heart is outlined by the calcium deposits. Other less common causes are virus infection, rheumatism or deep x-ray therapy. Treatment is surgical removal of the constricting scar tissue.

13

Coronary care

Death from coronary thrombosis is often due to arrhythmias—ventricular fibrillation, asystolic arrest, heart block or rapid tachycardia. In many patients in whom these fatal arrhythmias occur, the damage to the heart muscle is slight. In many other patients there are severe symptoms of heart failure, for example, those due to pulmonary oedema, which will respond to vigorous treatment, and, after recovery leave the patient with little disability and able to earn his living normally (see page 25). The recognition of the emergency threatening life in these circumstances, is a matter for constant vigilance aided by suitable monitoring systems. With only four minutes to restore the circulation if the heart stops, there is no time for 'sending for the doctor'. Lives are saved by the staff on the spot knowing what to do.

The coronary care ward has been introduced to meet this situation. The purpose of this special type of ward is to provide an environment with apparatus designed to detect cardiac emergencies, equipment to remedy them, and a staff trained in this special type of nursing.

As the patients in this ward are particularly likely to need emergency attention, a much larger number of nurses is needed per bed than on a general medical ward. Furthermore these wards need much more space round the beds than is usual. The ward becomes difficult to manage if there are more than four or six beds under the care of a single team. As emergencies occur as often by night as by day, it is essential that the cover at night is by fully trained nurses. The nursing on these wards is exacting but exciting and deeply interesting. A period on an intensive care ward should be included in the training of every nurse just as 'specialing' (i.e. a single seriously ill patient having a nurse do nothing but care for him) used to be part of the experience of every trained nurse. Specialing, in fact, has been replaced by the intensive care ward, largely as a result of the increased complexity of monitoring methods and the shortage of nurses.

Before describing the nursing of a coronary care ward (also referred to as coronary care unit, intensive care ward or unit and intensive therapy unit), the main pieces of apparatus may be briefly described. Most of them are described in greater detail at the end of the book.

APPARATUS

Beds

The bed in an intensive care unit is usually specially made. There are no springs, the base of the bed being a firm sheet of wood and the mattress of rubber or plastic foam. This has two purposes: the firm base allows external cardiac massage to be performed without moving the patient, and the absence of springs allows a portable x-ray set to be used in an emergency without delay.

By suitable screws, the top and bottom of the bed may be tilted up or down so that the patient's position can be changed from head up to head down, or up both ends or up in the middle and down both ends. Unfortunately, the mechanism for moving the bed in this way is usually of metal and interferes with the use of an x-ray screening set. This means that a separate bed with an entirely wooden base and foam mattress may be also needed for use with the x-ray set for inserting catheters. In all beds in an intensive care unit, the bed rail and mattress should be high enough to allow the x-ray set to pass beneath them.

X-ray screening sets

The most useful x-ray screening set is a 6″ portable image intensifier. This consists of an x-ray tube mounted at the bottom of a suitable framework so that it can be wheeled in under the bed. The x-ray beam is projected vertically upwards through the mattress and the patient to an image intensifier. This senses the shadows cast by the patient's body. From the intensifier tube, the impulses are taken by a cable to a television screen where they can be seen by the team who are inserting a pace-making catheter.

Oscilloscopes

The essential monitoring equipment is an oscilloscope for displaying the patient's electrocardiogram. In most intensive care wards there is an oscilloscope by the bed and a second one at the nurses' station. Here the electrocardiograms of all the patients being maintained are shown on a large oscilloscope. Most sets incorporate some sort of warning device, which will come on if the heart stops or goes too quickly or too slowly. This is usually an audible alarm signal, with, in most cases, a warning light. The patient is connected to the monitor either by the usual metal plates attached to the limbs by rubber armlets, or by small plates stuck to the chest by adhesive. In both cases an electrode jelly is usually used between the plate and the skin to maintain a moist contact—the dry skin is a good insulator and will prevent the voltage of the electrocardiogram being transmitted to the monitor.

Pacemakers

A pacemaker is necessary for maintaining the heart beat in some cases, usually in patients with heart block. Pacemakers may be for external or internal pace making.

External pacing. In external pacing, a plate electrode about 3 cm across is attached to the skin over the apex of the heart, and a second electrode is placed over the sternum or on the right side of the chest. Both electrodes have to be liberally covered with electrode jelly to allow an electric current to pass between them. The pacemaking machine is turned to a suitable voltage, usually about 20 to 30 volts, and to a suitable rate, say 70 beats per minute. When the machine is switched on, short electrical pulses of the selected voltage and rate pass between the plates, stimulating the heart to beat. It is possible to keep a heart going with this kind of pacing for days if a pacemaking catheter cannot be used, but it may be exhausting for the patient. This is because the electrical pulse passing through the chest stimulates all the muscles in its path, so that the muscles of the chest wall twitch each time the machine stimulates the heart.

Internal pacing. Internal pacing is commonly referred to as endocardial pacing, as the electrodes are in contact with the endocardium, the lining of the heart. The pacemaking catheter usually used for temporary pacemaking is a smooth flexible plastic coated wire. At one end are two platinum electrodes, one at the tip of the catheter and the second 1 cm from the tip. At the other end are two metal connections for connecting to the pacemaker. There are two sizes in common use, 6F (2 mm diameter) and 5F (1·7 mm diameter). The catheter is passed to the heart from a vein in the arm or neck, either by cutting down or by insertion through a special percutaneous

introducer. The tip of the catheter is lodged in the apex of the right
ventricle if the ventricle is to be paced, or against the atrial wall if
the atrium is to be paced. The pacemaking voltage usually needed
in the ventricle is 1 to 3 volts. In the atrium more may be required.

Pacemakers for use with endocardial pacing catheters are of
several types. There are large machines operated by mains electricity
and/or batteries and there are all sizes down to battery operated
machines little bigger than a matchbox, which can be taped to the
patient's arm. Many of them can be set so that they stop pacing if
the heart starts beating normally, but switch themselves on automatically if the heart stops or goes more slowly than the speed the
pacemaker is set for. This method of pacing is called *demand pacing*.

Defibrillators

A defibrillator is the next piece of equipment needed in an intensive
care ward. It is used to revert ventricular fibrillation and other
arrhythmias to sinus rhythm. The instrument may be one of two
types. The AC (alternating current) defibrillator works from the
mains. It is essentially a transformer with a switching arrangement
which allows a short pulse of AC current at a selected voltage to be
passed between two applicators. The DC (direct current) defibrillator
is a mains or battery operated machine. It consists of a large condenser which is charged up with electrical energy measured on a dial
in Joules or Watt-seconds. The charging up usually takes a few
seconds and there is usually a signal light to indicate when the
charge is ready. On pressing a switch the electrical energy is discharged between the plates. Some machines have a second switch
usually labelled 'discharge', which releases the charge on the
condenser *without passing it through the patient*. This is a safety
measure, as the accidental discharge of one of these machines
through a normally beating heart, may make the heart's ventricles
fibrillate. If the machine is left charged up, medical or nursing staff
may be accidentally killed while handling it. *The machine should
always be discharged by this switch after use.* If no switch is provided
it should be discharged on a specially made discharge plate or a
slightly damp towel folded on a non-conducting surface. Most units
are now equipped with the DC type of defibrillator.

The applicators for defibrillators are of several types, but all consist
of a pair of large metal plates with heavily insulated handles. The
metal may be a smooth plate of stainless steel or a sheet of woven
stainless steel gauze. There is often a safety feature to prevent

5

accidental discharge and ensure firm application to the chest wall. This is commonly a pressure switch so arranged that *pressing the applicator firmly down makes the switch contact.* This may be present in one or both applicators. There is usually a press button on one of the applicators for switching the defibrillation current on. In some machines this switch is on the machine, which has the disadvantage that it is almost impossible for one person to work it as two hands are needed to apply the applicators to the chest wall.

The instrument should be ready at all times with the applicators connected. When needed the applicators are first coated with a generous layer of electrode jelly, which should *completely* cover the metal which comes in contact with the patient. The defibrillator is switched to charge and when ready, one applicator is pressed *firmly* over the apex of the heart and the other placed over the right nipple or right anterior axillary line. The defibrillating switch is then pressed and the patient should give a convulsive twitch as the current passes. The ECG trace will disappear off the oscilloscope for a moment or two and then return. If the trace does not show reversal to a satisfactory state, the shock should be repeated with an increased charge. Several shocks may be needed. If there is no jerk from the patient when the defibrillate switch is pressed, then the machine is not working, the patient is completely paralysed by drugs or, by far the most likely, the applicator pressure switches were not on because the pressure was not firm enough. While one person can perform defibrillation safely, it is safer for two people to do this, each holding one applicator. There is always a slight risk of passing the defibrillation current through the operator instead of the patient if one person holds both applicators. If this happens, the result may be two people in urgent need of defibrillation instead of one.

After use the applicators should be cleaned with copious use of warm soapy water, as the electrode jelly contains enough electrolytes to corrode most grades of stainless steel rendering them non-conducting.

THE APPLICATORS SHOULD NEVER BE APPLIED DRY TO THE SKIN.

The defibrillating discharge is made at about 1,500 volts and will cause severe burns to the patient if the skin is dry. Similarly **never** place the applicators face to face and make a discharge. Dangerous sparking will occur and the gauze ones will be blasted full of holes. For demonstrating the use of the defibrillator, the applicators should be placed side by side on a special discharge plate or a *slightly* moistened folded towel.

These three pieces of equipment, *the monitoring oscilloscope*, the *pacemaker* and the *defibrillator* are the essential tools of the coronary care ward. Their use has been described in some detail as it is essential that everyone working in coronary care is thoroughly familiar with their use.

Suckers

Other pieces of equipment have more general applications. A sucker is used for removing fluid which accumulates in the trachea either as a result of left heart failure or infection. Its use is described in the section on surgical intensive care.

Electronic thermometers

An electronic thermometer is often used to measure the body temperature. The sensitive element is mounted on the end of a long cable and may be placed in the rectum. Temperature is recorded on a dial or on an oscilloscope. There is usually a simple method for checking the instrument.

Manometers

Pressure measurement may also be recorded.

Venous pressure. The venous pressure is most easily measured by a simple saline manometer. This is simply a length of plastic tubing connected to a polythene tube introduced into the right atrium from a vein. In some circumstances the left atrial pressure may be measured in the same way. The left atrial pressure is a more useful measurement, as it gives a good idea of the balance of the actions of the right and left ventricles and of the state of things in the lungs. Any rise in LAP will give early warning that the left ventricle is failing and that pulmonary congestion and oedema are impending.

Venous pressures can also be measured by transducers. With low pressure measurements, however, the method requires very experienced staff if reliable measurements are to be made even over short periods. Unless the staff of the recovery unit have a great deal of experience in the use of the transducers, the venous pressures are best measured with the simple saline tube.

Systemic pressure may also be measured by a catheter inserted into an artery. The simplest device for this measurement is the aneroid manometer specially adapted to allow measurement through a saline filled tube. A more expensive method is the use of a transducer of the type used in the operating theatre or at diagnostic catheterization. This can be arranged to show the pressure on the oscilloscope with the ECG or on a meter where the pressure can be read off.

Infusion apparatus

Infusion apparatus of various kinds is found in intensive care units. The simplest is the conventional bottle of blood or electrolyte solution, connected to the patient by tubing and drop chamber with an adjustable clamp to regulate the rate of flow. For some infusions greater accuracy is needed in the rate of delivery. This may be achieved by the use of a variety of electric gadgets which work by counting the drips and automatically adjusting the flow rate. A different method of infusion is by a small roller pump similar to that used for pumping blood in a heart lung machine. Here the rate of infusion depends upon the rate of rotation of the rollers and the size of the infusion tubing being squeezed by the rollers. Very precise adjustment of the distance between the rollers and the anvil against which they squeeze the tubing, is necessary.

Ventilators

Ventilators is the slightly misleading name for machines which maintain respiration. The name, however, precisely describes their function. They ventilate the lungs of patients who are too weak to breathe adequately, by blowing the lungs up and letting them down again. The machine is connected to either a tracheostomy or an endotracheal tube. The care of the trachea of patients on these machines is of utmost importance and is described in the section on surgical intensive care.

Laboratory measurements may be made in the intensive care unit. These may include measurements of haemoglobin, blood volume, cardiac output, blood gas analysis and blood and urinary electrolytes.

This long list of pieces of apparatus could be extended even further, but the main items found on most intensive therapy units have been mentioned. Although the list may seem frighteningly complicated, the purpose of all these instruments is quite simple—to maintain the output of the heart and the ventilatory function of the lungs. In the use of all these machines, it is important to remember that none of them replaces the need for vigilance on the part of the nursing staff, and no monitor is as good or tells as much as the appearance of the patient tells the doctor or nurse. The monitor, whatever its type, gives information about a single aspect of the patient only.

USE OF THE APPARATUS

If the nurse in an intensive care unit is to make intelligent use of the apparatus in it, she must know what the apparatus is being used for, how to control it and in what circumstances she must take immediate action. The action taken may be the immediate application of external cardiac massage or the calling of a doctor. We must first consider the monitoring equipment and its shortcomings (see Chapter 15).

The monitoring oscilloscope

The controls and general working of a typical *monitor* are described on page 126. It consists essentially of an oscilloscope on which millivolt changes are displayed. In the example described, there is also a ratemeter for giving a continuous recording of heart rate and an alarm signal which will sound if the rate recorded moves outside limits set on the dial showing the rate. In addition, each heart beat can be made to produce an audible bleep from the machine. The instrument can be coupled to a pace-maker, which will automatically take over and start pacing the heart if the rate falls below the limit set on the ratemeter dial. It sounds as if all the nurse has to do is retire to the office to which the information can be relayed, get out her knitting and make sure her cup of tea is freshly made. It doesn't work out like that.

PROBLEMS OF USE. 1. The first snag is that the noise made by the machine indicating the heart beats, sounds like a rather hefty new born chicken trying to find its mother. Four of them all going together at different rates makes an intensive care ward sound like an electronic farmyard. Add to this, say, two patients on ventilators and one patient on continuous suction, and the impression that the farmer is feeding the pigs and has turned on the milking machine is a strong one. A very short experience of this cacophony will drive most patients and all nurses to distraction.

The audible warning and bleeping heart beat are extremely useful on occasions—for example when the staff are heavily engaged with an emergency in one patient and have another who may also be in sudden trouble. The warning system can then be made audible, so that if anything goes wrong with the patient who is not the centre of attention, the trouble can be quickly recognized. At most other times the warning light is preferable.

2. A second major problem with any electrocardiographic monitoring system is the nonspecific nature of the electrocardiogram. Any muscle produces a voltage change when it contracts. If the patient moves about in bed and the muscles which he moves are between the points at which the ECG electrodes are attached, the machine will record the movement. This may cause the machine to record spurious heart beats and so give an alarm signal. To overcome this, most machines have a time factor built in so that the alarm will not sound unless the abnormal rate continues for several seconds, but in a restless patient this may not prevent false alarms. It is usually possible to avoid this source of bother by attaching the electrodes along the sternum, but this may be impossible, for example if the sternum is covered by surgical dressings.

A different alarm may sound if one of the ECG leads becomes disconnected. This will either cause the recording to stop in which case the machine will sound an alarm indicating cardiac arrest, or a violent oscillation may occur and be recorded as tachycardia. Here the cure is simple—connect up the leads.

These false alarms all mean that the machine is fallible. The first thing to do when any alarm is given is to look at the patient. If he appears to be all right, then try to decide whether the ECG tracing indicates a genuine change in heart action or merely something upsetting the recorder. If the latter, check the leads and connections to the machine including the plug to the mains if there is one.

Pacemakers

Pacemakers give surprisingly little trouble. If a patient on a temporary pacemaker stops pacing, the heart will usually continue to beat at the ventricular rate of 30–50 beats a minute after an initial pause of 15–30 seconds, during which an Adams-Stokes attack may occur. If it does not beat again spontaneously and cardiac arrest persists, external cardiac massage may be needed to keep the circulation going. The usual reason for pacemaker failure is that one of the leads to the machine has become disconnected. These should be checked. If the leads are all right at the pacemaker, and pacing has stopped, failure to pace in these circumstances is usually due to the tip of the pacemaker catheter moving from its position in the ventricle. This may be due to the heart's action—the catheter may be moved up into the outflow of the right ventricle, into the coronary sinus or down into the liver. Occasionally the catheter has been pulled back out of the heart by some movement of the patient. Sometimes this is easily recognized because the patient has reverted to heart block while the chest muscles have begun to twitch in time with the pacemaker. If both ends of the pacemaking catheter are in the correct position, then the failure may be due to a break in the catheter wire, or to the catheter tip failing to stimulate because it is in contact with unresponsive myocardium. Both these faults need to be treated by insertion of a new pacemaking catheter.

If the pacemaker itself is suspect it is easily tested. Attach a pacemaking catheter or a pair of wires to its terminals and set it to 4 or 6 volts. Place the other end of the wires on the tip of your tongue about 1 cm apart. You should feel a slight pricking sensation each time the pacemaker makes a pulse. If testing an internal/external machine make sure it is set to 4 volts on the *internal* range of voltage. A pulse of 40 volts through the tip of the tongue is not pleasant. This test can also be used to test a pacemaking catheter, but is usually unnecessary—a faulty catheter is best handed to an electronics technician for testing. A machine, however, may have to be tested in an emergency when a technician is not available.

Manometers

Pressure measurement is another monitoring procedure where the techniques appear frighteningly complicated to any nurse seeing them for the first time. In fact, the causes of failure or of error are usually very simple and obvious to anyone who is prepared to look for them. Faults in the electronic side of the measurement are unusual. Most of the difficulties are due to leaks, bubbles, or clots in the tubing of the manometer system.

Leaks can usually be avoided by using plastic tubing with junctions which lock together. The nurse must understand the system used and how it fits together, since if a leak does develop, rapid action may be needed to prevent serious trouble. Most systems are provided with 3-way taps so that saline can be flushed through the system. The nurse should examine each type of tap in use since the handles of the taps do not always point the same way. All manometers are connected to the patient by tubes filled with liquid, so that the position of the manometer will affect the pressure recorded. Raising the manometer will lower the measured pressure, lowering it will increase it by the weight of the vertical column of fluid (see page 134). All junctions, particularly on arterial systems should be inspected for leaks regularly. If a low pressure system such as venous pressure is monitored, remember that raising the pressure head may result in a *negative* pressure in the recording tubing. This can easily happen if the recording head is placed for convenience on the pillow of the bed. If the bed position is changed to head up, the pressure in the recording tubing may become negative. Any leak in this part of the system will now suck air into the recording tubing and instead of an obvious leak of blood or saline, there may be a very dangerous entry of air into the recording system. If the pressure is low enough, this air may pass into the patient's venous system causing air embolism.

Bubbles of air in the recording system will have different effects depending on the system used. In a saline manometer they will cause false high readings, since the air does not weigh but holds the saline column at a false level.

In an aneroid system, bubbles will not affect the recording of pressure unless they are large, when the movement of the aneroid needle will be less than it should be.

In an electronic transducer system, the volume changes are so small that any bubble will absorb the changes due to the blood pressure and a straight line recording of about the mean pressure will appear.

Getting rid of bubbles. These must **NOT** be flushed into the patient. When the bubble is in the tubing between the tap connecting the flushing saline to the pressure measuring system, great care is necessary since the air can easily be flushed into the patient. A sterile syringe should be connected to the tap and the bubble drawn back into the syringe. The tube is then refilled with saline and the tap turned to disconnect the saline.

When the bubble lies between the tap and the recorder, the procedure depends upon the type of manometer. A saline manometer may be allowed to overflow until the bubble is out of the tubing. An aneroid should be disconnected from the tap and the filling procedure for the saline part of the instrument repeated. An electronic transducer should be carefully flushed by opening the bleed cock on the transducer and running saline through it from the reservoir. **NEVER** apply forced suction or pressure to these electronic transducers, as the metal membrane may be seriously damaged.

Clots are uncommon with most types of manometer tubing now in use. However, if blood comes into contact with metal it is likely to clot. All 3-way taps should be plastic and blood should not be allowed to come into contact with the electronic pressure head in which there is a metal diaphragm. With occasional flushing most pressure measuring systems will function for days. Remember, however, that fluid flushed through the catheter is added to the patient, and should be recorded. The quantities should not be large in an adult, but may be significant in an infant or young child.

We may end this description of instruments and their short-comings with some pointers on how to handle recording failure. It might seem that this is more properly the province of the doctor or cardiological technician, but on most units the nursing staff find that dealing with failures are well within their capacity.

Fault	Cause	Remedy
No trace on oscilloscope	*a.* Machine is disconnected from mains	Plug it in
	b. Mains or machine is switched off	Switch it on
	c. Sweep is off the the screen	Adjust knob for 'Y' axis
	d. Machine broken	Get another
No electrocardiogram	*a.* ECG control set to O or calibrate	Switch to I, II, or III
	b. Lead has come out of machine or patient's contact plate	Reconnect it
ECG shows gross AC interference	*a.* Patient's contacts are dry	Apply fresh electrode jelly
	b. A patient's lead is disconnected	Connect it
	c. Someone is touching the patient	Hands off
	d. Electrode plates are dirty	Clean with metal polish
	e. Interference from other equipment	May have to put up with it, but all apparatus should be fitted with suppressors to stop this happening
No pressure record	*a.* Air bubble in tubing or recording head	Remove them

Fault	Cause	Remedy
	Tubing is acutely kinked	Straighten it. If kink is out of sight inside the patient, the tube will appear blocked. Try gently pulling out a cm or two
	c. Clot in tubing	Try flushing or cleaning with a stylette if a doctor advises it
	d. The end of the tubing is blocked by the vessel wall	In this circumstance it is easy to inject saline but impossible to aspirate, as the block is like a non-return valve. Withdraw the tubing slightly
	e. The end of the tube is in a small collapsed vein	Requires repositioning by doctor using a guide wire

The major part of this chapter has been devoted to the instruments used for intensive care. This is because the use of these is unfamiliar to nurses who have worked in a conventional ward. Even in general wards, however, monitors are being used with increasing frequency and their advantages and limitations must be more and more the concern of people working with them. No accumulation of gadgets, however, replaces the value of the nurse's observation of her patients and her sympathy with and care for the sick. Very few sick people get encouragement and hope from listening to the buzzings and bleepings of a machine. This must come from the words and bearing of the staff. The staff must be confident they understand their environment if they are to give their patients confidence. If that environment includes electronic monitors, then the staff must have a clear idea of what these monitors do.

The purpose of the intensive care ward will be apparent from what has already been considered in this book. Maintaining the cardiac output, the blood pressure, and the lung function are the basis of it. From these stems the maintenance of the function of the brain, kidney, liver and gut. Not every patient can be saved. Some arrhythmias and types of cardiac arrest will not respond to treatment. Sometimes the circulation can only be maintained in circumstances impossible for some other function. For example, in a failing heart the venous pressure may rise so high that the flow of urine ceases and uraemia develops. Urine will not flow if the perfusion pressure in the renal glomeruli falls below 60 mm Hg. If the arterial pressure after a cardiac infarct falls to 80 mm Hg while the venous pressure rises to 30 mm Hg urine cannot form. However, if the patient can be tided over this period by intensive care, including if necessary renal dialysis until the heart recovers its function, the patient may recover and return to active life.

The essentials of the treatment are simple. If the heart stops, maintain the circulation by external massage and maintain respiration while taking appropriate measures to get it going again. If the heart goes too fast to work efficiently, slow it down. If the heart goes too slowly to work efficiently, speed it up. Maintain ventilation by keeping the airways clear and the lungs free of oedema. Relieve pain and anxiety.

14

Cardiac surgical nursing

PREAMBLE

The quality of post-operative nursing has an immediate and profound importance to the patient who has just had a heart operation. Whilst it is usually true to say that the immediate survival of the patient depends on the right operation being done well by the surgical and anaesthetic team in the operating room, it remains true that prolonged survival depends on the skill and devotion of the team who look after the patient when the operation is over. This team consists of nursing, anaesthetic and surgical members and each group has a specific and well defined series of tasks to perform.

Cardiac surgical nursing is highly skilled and demands a high degree of care and attention to detail, yet it is not divorced from general nursing practices. The nurse in the team does her part by carrying out basic nursing techniques. These techniques and the ways in which they are used are best learned at the bedside under the tuition of an experienced sister, and it is not the purpose of this chapter to try and change this method of learning but to provide basic understanding of the reasons underlying the schemes of care.

All cardiac surgical nursing should be done in the intensive care ward. Ideally, this should be situated very close to the operating theatre and on the same floor level. Only in an intensive care ward devoted to cardiac surgical nursing is it possible to have the numbers of nursing staff and the equipment necessary to cope with the problems involved. It is essential that the nurses should be fully committed to their patient and that they should not be distracted by having to cope with minor details of ward administration, and answering the telephone.

THE PROBLEMS INVOLVED IN THIS TYPE OF NURSING

Any patient who undergoes cardiac surgery presents FOUR types of problem in the early post-operative period. These are:

1. Haemorrhage
2. Shock
3. Pain and apprehension
4. Problems involved in supplying physiological demands.

We shall discuss each of these in greater detail, both from the point of view of detection and of treatment, but first it is necessary to describe and account for the various items of equipment, the observations which have to be made and the charts which have to be kept on a typical patient who has had a cardiac operation. As the description develops, it will be useful to keep each of the above problems in mind. The description will be that of the care given to a patient who has undergone major cardiac surgery. Some patients will have undergone lesser procedures and the intensive care regime may then be modified. Broadly speaking, the full regime is applied to every patient who has undergone 'open' cardiac surgery, i.e., that surgery performed when the heart is not supporting the circulation. A less intensive regime is usually applied to patients who have had 'closed' cardiac surgery. Obviously, the full regime will be given to a patient who has tolerated a closed procedure poorly.

THE USUAL ROUTINE OF INTENSIVE CARE

The patient is placed on his bed in the operating theatre. The bed should be warm as some of these patients have a subnormal temperature at this time. The patient rests upon a ripple mattress with the head and shoulders and the feet slightly elevated. An *endotracheal tube* has been passed before operation and this is left in position afterwards in order to ventilate the patient by a *positive pressure ventilator*. A *urinary catheter*, also passed before operation drains into a calibrated measuring flask. A cannula lies in an artery, usually the radial artery at the wrist, and this will be used for measuring the *arterial blood pressure* and for taking arterial blood samples. A *blood infusion* runs into a vein in one or other of the upper limbs (Fig.31).

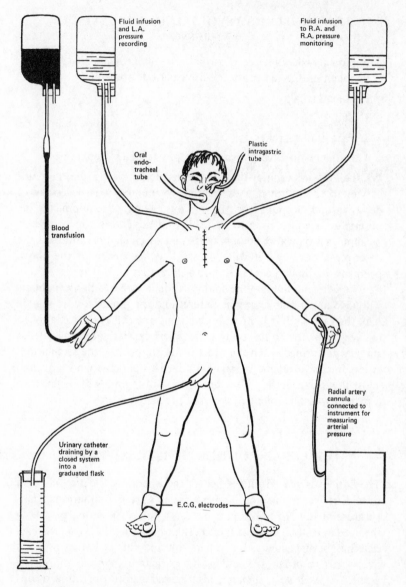

Fig.31. Diagram showing the various monitoring and other connections made for the full intensive nursing care regime.

Coming out of the chest wall by means of surgical incisions are two sorts of tubes. First, *drainage tubes*, carrying away blood which

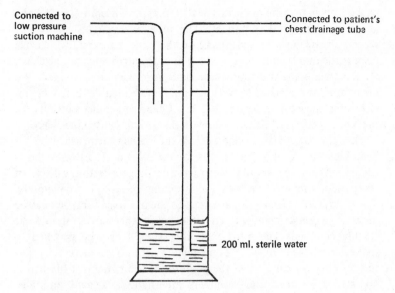

Connected to low pressure suction machine

Connected to patient's chest drainage tube

200 ml. sterile water

Fig.32. Diagram of underwater seal drainage system.

might collect around the heart and in the mediastinum. These pass to underwater seal bottles, which act as one way traps, preventing air entering the patient whilst at the same time, allowing blood and fluid out (Fig.32). Back in the ward, each drainage tube and its underwater seal are put on continuous suction at a low (-5 cm water) negative pressure. Each tube needs to be 'milked' frequently in order to prevent it becoming blocked by blood clots.

Atrial pressure recording

The other tubes to emerge directly from the patient's chest are the *cannulae* which are used to measure atrial pressures. These cannulae are fine bore plastic tubes which have been inserted into the atria when the operation has been in progress. Afterwards, each is brought out through the chest wall and connected to a drip set through which 5 per cent dextrose is infused slowly (Fig.35). A 3-way tap is inserted into this system, so that it is possible to put in a side tube open to the air and attached to an ordinary wooden school one foot ruler.

Most of the time, the 3-way tap system can work as an ordinary infusion set with the side arm occluded. If however, the side arm is opened into direct communication with the patient, the fluid will be pushed up it to a height which will represent (in cm of water) the atrial pressure of that patient. The base of the ruler should be placed always on the same mark on the patient's chest, which has been made at a level thought to be that of the atrium inside the chest. By this means the pressure inside both atria may be measured. We have found this method to be simpler and more reliable than using an electronic measuring device (Fig.35). Great care must be taken to prevent air entering either system as this would cause embolism.

Thus the patient is wheeled back to the intensive care ward on his bed. This time is most hazardous for the patient. The nurse who is accompanying him should do so with her fingers resting on one of the patient's femoral arteries and watching his colour very closely. The glass bottles which are attached to the drainage tubes should be guarded against breakage and the tubes themselves should be doubly clamped. The infusion bottles should also be watched to make sure that no air bubbles manage to get into the drip sets. Once in the intensive care ward, the position of the patient in the bed is adjusted. The head and shoulders are slightly elevated and also the feet. This position promotes venous drainage from the head and the feet. The endotracheal tube is attached to the tubes of the ventilator, which should have been checked for safety and proper functioning beforehand. On each limb, a conventional ECG electrode is placed and an ECG oscilloscope is thus connected. The urinary catheter is attached to a graduated flask, so that the rate of urine drainage can be measured. The motor of the ripple mattress is connected to the electricity supply and turned on.

Observations and charts

Three types of observations are recorded.

1. The arterial blood pressure, pulse rate and apex rate, and the atrial pressures are recorded quarterly hourly initially and less often later on. As these observations together give an indication of the heart's action, they are recorded on the same chart.

2. On a second chart, hourly recordings are made of the volume of urine passed into the graduated flask and of the volumes of non-blood fluids infused. Each 24 hour period is concluded by working out the grand totals.

3. On a third chart, record is made of the amount of blood lost down the chest drainage tubes and of the amount of blood given to the patient in the same period.

These are the basic three charts which provide information about the patient. To them may be added others to keep a record of drugs given from hour to hour and of changes in the biochemical investigation of the patient. These are a matter of choice for the individual nurse, but the basic three charts are the cardinal records of the patient's progress. Sometimes these are combined into one large master chart, but many people feel that confusion may arise when too much information is presented at one time on such a chart.

The ventilator

Nearly all patients who have had major heart surgery are placed on a ventilator afterwards. The reasons for this are two. First, the lungs are often difficult and stiff to inflate. To allow the patient to breathe spontaneously would require a great effort on his part and this would mean that the heart would have to work harder. Secondly, mechanical inflation of the lungs means that it can be safely assumed that the efficiency of breathing is satisfactory, thus removing an area of doubt when considering the condition of the patient. There are many types of ventilator, but we prefer a machine which is fairly simple to use and which delivers a constant chosen volume of gas to the patient at a predetermined number of times per minute. On the machine, pressure recording dials show the pressures needed to achieve this. We have not chosen to use pressure constant ventilators which may deliver a variable volume of gas to the patient's lungs, since in the presence of 'stiff' lungs, too little oxygen may be made available to the patient.

Before being attached to the patient, the ventilator is sterilized internally by the method recommended by the makers and is tested. Every 24 hours, the ventilator on any one patient is changed to a fresh clean one, so that the dangers of infection of the bronchial tree are reduced.

The ventilator usually contains a device to warm and to moisten the air being pumped into the patient's lungs. This is usually a form of heated water bath and the level of water in it and the temperature of that water must be checked occasionally.

All patients who have had open heart surgery require to breathe an oxygen enriched mixture and usually oxygen is added to the ventilator so that 50 per cent oxygen-air mixture is given to the patient. The effect of open heart surgery upon the lungs is to impair the diffusion of oxygen across the alveolar membrane and consequently a normal arterial oxygen saturation can only be achieved by the breathing of oxygen enriched air. The concentration of oxygen should never be allowed to exceed 50 per cent except for a few minutes, since any higher concentration *rapidly causes further lung damage.*

The efficiency of ventilation is measured by the estimation of the oxygen tension, carbon dioxide tension and pH of arterial blood. This is measured on special apparatus which should be kept in or near the intensive care ward. The blood sample is usually drawn from the indwelling cannula in the radial artery. The actual measurements are performed by a technician. In general terms, the rate and depth of ventilation are adjusted so that the partial pressure of carbon dioxide in the blood is maintained between 30–40 mm Hg. The amount of oxygen added is sufficient to achieve a partial pressure of oxygen of 100 mm Hg, providing that concentration of oxygen in the inspired air is not allowed to exceed 50 per cent.

Care of the endotracheal tube

With moderate doses of narcotics to maintain analgesia and sedation, nearly all patients easily tolerate an endotracheal tube. This is usually fixed in position by a tape which has been passed around the patient's neck. Nevertheless, some individuals cannot tolerate the tube and in these rare cases, a tracheostomy may be necessary.

The cuff of the endotracheal tube should be inflated with the minimum amount of air necessary to prevent an air leak around it. This amount is not a constant figure and usually the cuff pressure will be checked from time to time by the anaesthetist. *Too much pressure causes ischaemia and ulceration* of the tracheal mucosa and this is to be avoided at all costs.

Infection can easily enter the bronchial tree by way of the endotracheal tube. Accordingly, when sputum has to be removed from the trachea below the tube, suction is applied by the use of a sterile tube introduced into the trachea down the endotracheal tube in a sterile manner, by a masked nurse wearing disposable sterile plastic gloves. Every 24 hours, a sample of sputum is sent for full bacteriological examination.

The tube stops the patient from talking. This means distress in itself and the nurse can help the patient a great deal by talking to him. She should talk in normal tones and in such a way that the patient can answer by moving his head or eyes.

NORMAL COURSE IN THE INTENSIVE CARE WARD

Usually, the patient returns from the operating theatre in the late morning or early afternoon. The rest of the day sees a slow improvement in the appearance of the patient. The amount of blood draining from the chest diminishes rapidly and usually the patient will require drugs to abolish pain and maintain sedation. Ideally, all drugs given to the patient should be administered intravenously, as this ensures that the absorption into the blood stream is certain. The settings on the ventilator are adjusted according to the results of the arterial blood gas analysis. The nurse maintains constant observation on the vital signs noted above and she will also note that the skin slowly becomes warmer. On the morning following the operation, the interval between observations can be increased. The patient is allowed to breathe spontaneously, first through the endotracheal tube and then with the tube removed. A portable chest x-ray is taken and if this is normal, the chest drainage tubes are removed. If bowel sounds have been heard, the patient is allowed fluid by mouth and if this is tolerated, the amount is slowly increased so that intravenous fluids may be stopped. The left atrial cannula is usually removed early and the right atrial cannula may be left *in situ* for several days. The ECG leads are usually left attached to the patient for two days, so that any abnormality of rate or rhythm can be detected rapidly.

Finally, if the patient's condition permits, the urinary catheter and ECG leads are removed and all cannulae withdrawn from the patient. He is then allowed to return to the surgical ward from which he came. At this time, all drugs are given either orally or by intramuscular injection.

PROBLEMS OCCURRING IN THE INTENSIVE CARE WARD

If all patients progressed normally throughout the post-operative period, the need for intensive care would disappear. Problems may occur rapidly and dramatically, or they may creep up slowly so that the mentally relaxed observer may consider all is well. The purpose of the regime outlined above is to expose such problems as soon as they arise and having done this, the appropriate remedy may be applied.

Haemorrhage

Some bleeding always occurs from the heart and its surrounding tissues after a cardiac operation. Usually this diminishes rapidly.

In the early years of open cardiac surgery, the techniques and instruments used often caused damage to the blood, creating amongst other things a diminished clotting ability. Nowadays, such damage rarely occurs and the usual cause of bleeding is failure of the surgeon to identify a source of bleeding and stop it. This means that any patient who is considered to be bleeding excessively should be returned to the theatre immediately for *re-exploration* to find the bleeding point. The point at which bleeding becomes 'excessive' varies. Usually, a blood loss of 500 ml in 1 hour, or a loss of 300 ml in an hour for three consecutive hours, is considered to be excessive. Sometimes, faced with a comparatively rare blood group, the surgeon may decide to re-operate sooner. At the second operation, a bleeding point is often found and dealt with. Occasionally no source of bleeding is found in spite of the most careful search. In these circumstances, the haemorrhage usually ceases when the chest is closed a second time. Only if bleeding still persists is it fair to assume that a clotting deficit is present. The laboratory is then asked to perform investigations which will test the efficiency of the various stages of the clotting mechanism. Once identified, the appropriate treatment may be given.

As blood is lost in the drainage tubes then it will be necessary to replace it. Blood is given to the patient at such a rate and volume that the right or left atrial pressure is maintained at its normal level for that patient. The blood given should ideally be warmed to 37° C in a special water bath, and each unit of blood given to the patient should be accompanied by the slow intravenous injection of 5 ml of 10 per cent calcium chloride solution. This drug is given so that the citrate in the administered blood will not significantly affect the serum calcium concentration. If this concentration were to decrease, the action of the heart might be seriously affected.

Needless to say, all the routine precautions against giving the wrong type of blood to a patient are always observed, no matter how great the urgency.

When excessive haemorrhage is occurring, the nurse should be assiduous in her care of the chest drainage tubes. The amount of 'milking' needed to ensure that the tubes do not become blocked is increased and as the patient is returned to the theatre, it is wiser not to clamp the tubes, thus allowing no collection of blood around the heart. (Cardiac tamponade, see below.)

Shock or low output syndrome

Shock means widely different things to different people and this is the reason why so much difficulty is encountered by nurses in understanding it. Shock is the clinical state in which the cardiac output is insufficient to supply the metabolic needs of the tissues. For this reason, there is an increasing use of the more explicit *low cardiac output syndrome* instead of the older, less precise term.

The major function of blood flow to the tissues is to supply oxygen and nutrients to the cells and to remove carbon dioxide and other waste products. If the cardiac output falls below a certain level, then insufficient supply of oxygen and nutrients occurs and there is an accumulation of waste products. As a result of this impaired perfusion, two things happen.

1. The organ begins to lose its function.

2. The tissue cells change over to anaerobic respiration in order to supply energy. This is not nearly so efficient as aerobic respiration and leads to the accumulation of acids. These in turn cause acidosis.

In the early stages of the low cardiac output syndrome, physiological compensation occurs, so that the diminished cardiac output is directed towards two tissues preferentially. By vasoconstriction of the vessels in the viscera, muscles and skin, the blood flow to the brain and the myocardium is preserved. Unfortunately, this response, although beneficial to the patient in the short-term, produces further underperfusion of the rest of the tissues of the body and accordingly, makes worse the state of 'shock'.

CLINICAL PICTURE OF LOW CARDIAC OUTPUT SYNDROME. 1. The patient is pale and has a cold skin as a result of poor skin perfusion. Peripheral pulses may not easily be palpable.

2. The urinary output as measured in the graduated flask is small (below 30 ml per hour). These two features are due to underperfusion of tissues.

3. The arterial blood pressure is 'normal' or low and often the pulse is rapid. The definition of *low cardiac output syndrome* concerns volumes and flow of blood to the tissues. Whilst undoubtedly, the level of arterial blood pressure is important within certain wide

limits, say over 70 mm Hg systolic, the presence of a 'normal' pressure does not rule out the presence of low output syndrome, if at the same time, clinical evidence of poor tissue perfusion is present.

4. Analysis of the arterial blood will show a *low pH* and a high level of acid metabolic products, thus proving that some tissues at least are being underperfused by arterial blood.

If left untreated, the syndrome of low cardiac output often leads to the death of the patient. The accumulation of acids in the blood reduces the force with which the heart can expel blood and the intense vasoconstriction of the vessels in the muscles and viscera leads to severe hypoxic damage in those tissues. When this occurs, the clinical picture deteriorates rapidly.

CAUSES OF LOW CARDIAC OUTPUT SYNDROME. 1. Inadequate venous return (Oligaemia)

  a. due to low circulating blood volume (absolute oligaemia)

  b. due to vasodilatation, causing the volume of blood available to be too small to fill fully the increased volume of the vascular bed (relative oligaemia).

2. Failure of the heart to pump efficiently

a. Muscle causes

b. Valve causes

c. Pericardial causes.

1. OLIGAEMIA—CAUSES AND TREATMENT. If the volume of blood returning to the heart falls, then the pressure with which it distends the right atrium and ventricle is diminished. This leads to a fall in the output of blood into the left atrium and ventricle. In turn, the cardiac output is diminished and low output syndrome occurs.

The *pressure of distention* of the right atrium is measured by the *central venous pressure* recording and if low readings are obtained, then it is certain that the volume of blood in the circulatory system is not enough (Fig.31). 'Central venous pressure' is the right atrial pressure.

The first step in the diagnosis of the cause of low output syndrome is to measure the central venous pressure. If a measurement below 5 cm of water is obtained, then oligaemia is present and must be corrected. Infusion of blood, plasma or some other fluid will correct oligaemia and the choice of which depends on what it is thought that the patient has lost or needs most. The infusion can be as rapid as possible if a constant measurement of the central venous pressure is made.

On rare occasions oligaemia may be the result of a pathological vasodilatation. The result is that the capacity of the vascular system is increased and the volume of blood within the patient is no longer sufficient to produce a satisfactory venous pressure. The cardiac output thus falls and tissue perfusion suffers. Such states may occur in spinal injuries or septicaemia. Again, the mainstay of treatment is to infuse fluid in order to produce a normal venous pressure.

2. FAILURE OF THE HEART TO PUMP. The cardiac output may fall owing to inefficiency of the heart as a pump. Such inefficiency may begin in the valves, the myocardium or the pericardium.

a. The valves. Sudden damage to a normal valve, as occurs in infection or mechanical failure of a prosthetic valve will always lead to a poor cardiac output. When low output syndrome results from this cause, it is often fatal unless extremely rapid valve replacement is performed.

b. The myocardium. Low output syndrome resulting from a damaged myocardium is the most common complication of heart surgery. The damage may be chronic, having occurred as a consequence of valvular or coronary artery disease, or it may be acute, as a result of surgical trauma. After cardiac surgery, damaged myocardium may lead to low output syndrome in one of two ways:

 a. By the poor power of contraction,

 b. By various dysrhythmias (disorders of rhythm).

The dysrhythmias are dealt with elsewhere in this book, but some features which are pronounced in surgical patients should be stressed. Possibly the most common arrhythmia is the ventricular ectopic beat. If untreated, then ventricular tachycardia and ventricular fibrillation may follow. It has been shown that ventricular ectopic beats occur much more frequently in the presence of a low serum potassium level (below 4·7 M Eq/L). Now the cardiac surgical patient is almost always suffering from potassium deficiency before surgery. This usually is caused by potassium-losing diuretics and the effect of the low serum potassium is enhanced by the digoxin which most severe cardiac patients receive. After surgery, therefore, the serum potassium is frequently measured and steps taken to elevate it if necessary. It is certain that attention paid to the level of serum potassium will result in the abolition of most ventricular ectopics and unexpected ventricular fibrillation. Recently, the importance of the serum potassium in patients with coronary artery disease has become increasingly recognized.

c. *The pericardium.* The inevitable loss of blood into the pericardium after heart surgery is usually small in amount and drains quickly into the chest drains. Occasionally however, it may accumulate in the pericardial sac and not drain away. In these circumstances, the pressure within the pericardium increases and ultimately interferes with the full relaxation and filling of the heart. The cardiac output falls and low output syndrome results. This condition is called cardiac tamponade (see page 87). It is characterized clinically by a falling cardiac output in the presence of a rising central venous pressure. In addition, if right and left atrial pressures are being monitored, they rapidly approximate to give the same readings. Cardiac tamponade may occur even if the pericardium is left widely open at surgery. Suspicion of its onset may be aroused when intermittent large losses of blood from the chest drains are separated by very low amounts.

THE MANAGEMENT OF LOW OUTPUT SYNDROME. *a. Diagnosis.* If minute to minute measurement of cardiac output were available in the ward, the diagnosis would present no difficulty. At the moment, however, we have to rely on indirect assessments of cardiac output. The most important signs are the colour and warmth of the skin and the rate of urine production. The level of the arterial pressure is of less importance, providing it is above 80 mm Hg systolic. The presence of inadequate perfusion of the tissues may be detected by increasing metabolic acidosis of the arterial blood. We emphasize again the importance of skin warmth and urine production. A patient with a warm skin and a good production of urine and with an arterial blood pressure of 80/60 mm Hg has a much better cardiac output than a patient with an arterial pressure of 120/80 mm Hg and cold skin and no urine production. The failure to detect the presence of low cardiac output because of a 'normal' arterial pressure, is one of the most common yet unforgivable mistakes made in the intensive care ward.

b. Treatment of low cardiac output syndromes. If the patient is not being mechanically ventilated already, then this is started. The inspired oxygen concentration is adjusted to a level of 50 per cent. By this means, the work of respiration is taken from the patient and optimum oxygenation is achieved. Small doses of narcotics, either diamorphine (2 mg) or omnopon (5 mg) given as necessary by intravenous injection, will stop the patient 'fighting' the ventilator.

c. *Correction of oligaemia.* The right and left atrial pressures are then measured. Usually, the left has a higher pressure indicating partial left ventricular failure, but sometimes the right will be higher, showing partial failure of the right ventricle. It is our practice to measure both, but to place particular emphasis on the higher of the two. If the left atrial pressure is the higher, plasma is infused to bring it up to about 25 cm of water. This is the optimum level to which the left atrial pressure may be elevated without causing pulmonary oedema. Occasionally, the right atrial pressure is higher and infusions should be controlled to bring it between 10 and 15 cm of water.

These manoeuvres will successfully treat many cases of low output syndrome. If unsuccessful, then it may be assumed that the cause is cardiac. Careful listening to the heart may detect a faulty valve, but usually valvular causes of low cardiac output are ruled out. The type and rate of drainage of blood from the chest is assessed in order to rule out cardiac tamponade.

Scrutiny of the charts may be needed to detect the rising venous or atrial pressure which will occur when cardiac tamponade begins. Such is the fear of cardiac tamponade in any patient with low output syndrome that it may be diagnosed incorrectly in a patient not responding to other measures. The cardinal features of tamponade should be present before a diagnosis is made. The only treatment for cardiac tamponade is to reopen the chest and remove the blood clot. Fiddling around with drains and washing tubes out with saline is ineffective, time wasting and dangerous.

Usually, however, low output is the result of myocardial damage. If any dysrhythmias are occurring, they are abolished by the appropriate treatment. Any metabolic acidosis, which causes a further deterioration in myocardial performance, is measured and accurately corrected. The intense vasoconstriction of the skin may be assumed to be also present in the viscera. As explained, this is damaging and prejudices the patient's recovery. Accordingly, we usually give a vasodilator to overcome this. Our drug of choice is largactil 50 mg iv, and if that does not work, as evidenced by increase in skin temperature and an increased urine production, then we give hydrocortisone 150 mg per Kg body weight iv. Only rarely have we had to use the α blocking agent, phenoxybenzamine. When a vasodilator works, it will be necessary to infuse blood or plasma so as to maintain the atrial pressures.

d. Use of drugs. If it is thought that the cardiac output is still abnormally low, then drugs may be given which enhances the power of contractility of the myocardium.

They are:

a. Calcium chloride

b. Isoprenaline

c. Adrenalin.

CALCIUM CHLORIDE. This drug is given iv in 5 ml dose of the 10 per cent solution. In enhancing cardiac action, it may cause irritability as shown by ventricular ectopic beats, as may all three drugs.

ISOPRENALINE. This drug speeds up the heart and also increases the power of contraction. Usefully, it is also a mild peripheral vaso-dilator. These three actions make Isoprenaline a most useful drug in the treatment of low output syndrome. Usually, we give a 0·01 mg test dose iv and if a satisfactory response is obtained, then we put 2 mg Isoprenaline in a 500 ml bottle of 5 per cent dextrose solution and infuse it iv at such a rate as to cause a tachycardia of 110 per minute. Usually, Isoprenaline improves skin perfusion and urinary output. The arterial blood pressure will also rise.

ADRENALIN. This drug is a useful cardiac stimulant but, unfortunately, causes peripheral vasoconstriction. We have tended to use it only on patients who have not responded to Isoprenaline and only then in conjunction with vasodilators to offset its peripheral effect. Again, we usually give a test dose of 1 ml of 1:100,000 solution and if the response is favourable, infuse slowly a solution of 2 ampoules of 1:1,000 solution in 500 ml of dextrose solution.

Most patients respond to the management outlined above. Some patients respond very poorly however, and the possibility of cardiac tamponade again arises. Unless one can say with complete confidence that it is not the cause of the problem, it is better to return the patient to theatre for exploration. The possible harm done by a negative exploration is far outweighed by the great advantage of relieving an unsuspected tamponade.

Relief of pain and apprehension

Pain suffered after a surgical operation is neither character improving nor necessary. With the use of the appropriate drugs given sufficiently frequently and by the correct route of administration, complete relief of pain is possible. If at the same time, the patient may be relieved of anxiety, a further benefit arises, because endogenous adrenaline released during fear may have disturbing effects on the cardiac rhythm.

We use either Omnopon in 5 mg doses or diamorphine in 2 mg doses to achieve analgesia and sedation. The drug chosen is given via the drip tubing into a vein. This ensures that it is absorbed into the blood stream and has a very rapid effect. If more analgesia or sedation is needed, the dose may be repeated every five minutes until the desired effect is achieved. In this way, the drug is 'titrated' into the patient and since every patient will vary in his pain threshold and consequent need for the drug, the nurse can be sure that the minimal effective amount of the drug is given. The bogey of respiratory depression does not occur because the patient is usually being mechanically ventilated. In any event, relief of pain will always be accomplished before depression of respiration ensues. For the reasons outlined above, we reject the normal practice of giving large doses of opiates intramuscularly at set time intervals. We believe that *no* patient should have pain after *any* surgical procedure. To allow pain to occur is both inhumane and medically dangerous. A patient who has pain which persists in spite of intravenous analgesia may have a low pain threshold. This does not mean he is of inferior moral calibre. The presence of pain will prevent coughing and this will lead to the accumulation of sputum with its serious consequences.

The only other drug which we use is phenoperidine in 2 mg doses and again by the intravenous route. This drug is used sparingly for those patients who seem to be suffering no pain and who are adequately sedated by opiates, yet who are tending to 'fight' the ventilator.

We have found no real use for drugs such as diazepam (Valium) in this period.

Problems involved in supplying physiological demands

1. FLUID BALANCE. All patients who undergo a thoracotomy suffer from some degree of ileus afterwards. This is especially true of patients after open heart surgery. Until bowel sounds are

heard in the patient's abdomen, a Levins tube passed into the stomach is aspirated hourly and fluids are given intravenously (Fig.31).

Our practice is to give the patient 1,500 ml of 5 per cent dextrose in water in the first 24 hours after operation. After that time, 2 litres of 5 per cent dextrose and 500 ml of normal saline are given in each 24-hour period. To this volume is added a volume of normal saline equivalent to the volume of gastric aspirate in the previous 24-hour period.

As soon as bowel sounds return, a small amount of fluid is passed into the stomach every hour via the Levins tube. If this seems to be tolerated, the amount given by this route is increased and the amount given by intravenous infusion diminished.

2. NUTRITION. As soon as bowel sounds return and fluid is absorbed, then it will be possible to maintain the nutrition of the patient. We have found that this is best achieved by the patient receiving normal ward diet. In an unconscious patient, this is liquidized by an electric mixer and is given at the appropriate times down the Levins tube. We rarely use proprietary brands of liquid food. Intravenous alimentation with soluble fats and amino acids only rarely has to be given.

15

Apparatus

THE SPHYGMOMANOMETER

The sphygmomanometer is the simplest instrument available for measuring arterial blood pressure. A flat inflatable rubber cuff about 4″ × 10″ (10 cm × 25 cm) in size, is contained in a strong arm-band. The cuff has two rubber tubes entering it, one for inflating and deflating it, the other for connecting to a pressure manometer by a simple metal connector. The manometer may be either a mercury column or an aneroid gauge.

Use of the sphygmomanometer

The arm-band is applied to the arm so that its lower edge is 6 cm or so above the elbow. It should be wound round with the bag applied first and placed to that the middle of the bag comes over the brachial artery on the medial (inner) aspect of the arm. The bag can be easily felt through the fabric of the arm-band. (If in doubt, inflate it.) The arm-band is then wound evenly round the bag and its end tied, either by tucking it in, or by hooking on to metal bars, or by plastic sticky fabric depending on the type. It is important that the application is even so that the rubber bag is held close to the arm over its whole length.

Now find the pulsation of the brachial artery at the elbow. With the other hand pump up the pressure by squeezing the rubber bulb, having first closed the valve by screwing it down (Fig.33). When the arterial pulse disappears, pump up the pressure to about 20 mm higher. Now apply the stethoscope chest piece to the place where the arterial pulse was felt and let the pressure down slowly. When blood starts to come through under the cuff, you should hear it as a series of soft thumping sounds in time with the heart. The point at which the sounds are first heard is the systolic pressure. Continue to let

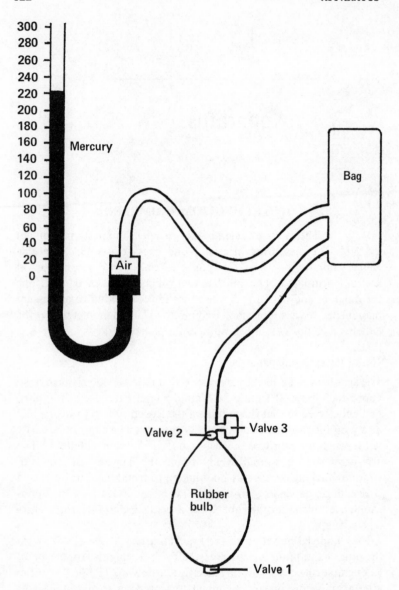

Fig.33. The sphygmomanometer. This is simply a mercury U-tube usually made with a reservoir on one side and a mercury column on the other. It connects to a rubber bag which is fixed to the arm by a linen cuff. The rubber bag is inflated by a rubber bulb which has two valves—one either side of it—so arranged that air will only pass through the bulb into the bag. The bag can be deflated by a screw valve placed between the bag and the bulb.

down the pressure and you should next find the sounds suddenly become softer. This is the diastolic pressure. Later at a lower pressure the sounds usually disappear. Suppose the sounds appeared at 120 mm Hg, become softer at 80 mm Hg and disappeared at about 45 mm Hg. This is usually recorded as 120/80 mm Hg. In some places it is usual to record the point of disappearance of the sounds, which would be written 120/80/45 mm Hg in this example.

COMPLICATIONS. The sequence of events is sometimes different to that just described. On some occasions the sounds disappear completely at the diastolic pressure and the point where the sound became softer is absent. Sometimes there is no sharp change, the sounds becoming progressively fainter until they disappear, making the diastolic pressure difficult to estimate. In some conditions the sounds are audible without an arm cuff being applied. This means that the diastolic pressure may have to be recorded as zero, if there is no obvious change in intensity to give a diastolic reading. Finally there is sometimes an important oddity called the *silent interval*. This is usually found in patients with high blood pressures and is particularly likely to occur if the sphygmomanometer cuff is let down very slowly. A typical recording with a silent interval occurs in the following way. The cuff may be pumped up to say 240 mm Hg and then allowed to deflate. The sounds are heard at, say, 220 mm Hg and continue to 180 mm Hg, when they disappear. If the cuff deflation is allowed to continue gently the sounds reappear at, say, 145 mm Hg, continue to 120 mm Hg and then disappear once more. It is very important to record this as a blood pressure of 220/120 mm Hg and not 220/180 mm Hg or 220/180/120 mm Hg. Occasional records of patients being treated for hypertension are made difficult to interpret, because the nurse recording the blood pressure has not understood the significance of the silent interval.

Lastly, if no sounds are audible do not necessarily blame your inexperience with the stethoscope. Even with a good quality diaphragm stethoscope, the sounds may be absent or very difficult to hear. If you can feel no pulse at the elbow there may be no sounds to hear, but if you can feel a pulse then the systolic pressure can be recorded at the point at which it appears on deflating the cuff.

ACCURACY OF MEASUREMENT. The accuracy of blood pressures recorded in this way is surprisingly high. The method depends upon producing a pressure under the arm-band which is the same as that in the bag. Provided the armlet is evenly applied and the arm not enormous, the pressure recorded by sphygmomanometry is the same as that obtained by intra-arterial measurement with an electronic pressure transducer. When the cuff is badly applied or the arm very big, the pressure recorded is too high, as the cuff has to be blown up tighter than should be necessary to squash the brachial artery flat. The accuracy of these measurements depends upon the manometer recording correctly. Two simple errors may invalidate measurements with the mercury type. The first is loss of mercury from the reservoir. The instrument should read O when on a level surface before the cuff is pumped up. If it does not, get the mercury reservoir checked. The second is recording with the instrument tilted. If this is done the pressure recorded will be too high, as the mercury column is in effect weighing the pressure in the cuff. In general, place the instrument on a level surface and see it stays level during measurement.

The aneroid manometer is not subject to errors of the type just described, and is a simple and accurate instrument. The oscillations of the needle which occur as the pressure is dropped, make it a little more difficult to decide on the systolic and diastolic pressures, but with practice the results are as consistent as those obtained by the mercury type.

THE ELECTROCARDIOGRAPH

The electrocardiograph is a recording voltmeter. The usual machines, once connected up, are simple to use. They may be mains or battery operated.

Use of the electrocardiograph

The machine should be switched on to allow it to warm up. While it is warming up the contact plates are placed on the arms and legs. These plates may be covered with fabric, in which case they should be wet with water, or metal, in which case they are moistened with electrode jelly. They are attached by perforated rubber straps. The straps should be firm but not tight. The patient's cables are then attached to the plates. It is important to get them on the correct limbs. The leads are usually marked with letters and are also coloured. Unfortunately, machines of more than a year or two old may have a colour code different from that given below. The present colouring is used on some machines with no letters:

Colour	Letters	Limb
Red	R A	Right arm
Yellow	L A	Left arm
Black	R L	Right leg
Green	L L	Left leg
White	P L	Chest lead

The white lead is attached to a small sucker. This sucker is attached to the chest.

The machine is now warmed up and may be standardized. It is switched to run and the paper should run out at the standard speed of 25 mm per second. A 1 millivolt pulse is put into the ECG with the selector switch set at O, cal or test by a switch for the purpose and the deflection adjusted to 1 cm. Between each adjustment the paper is stopped. A momentary pressure on the switch is all that is needed. If the calibration voltage is maintained by prolonged depression of the switch, most machines will not hold the deflection. The trace will begin to drift to the O line and deflect beyond zero when the switch is turned off. An adjusting knob is available on most machines to adjust the response to the test voltage. On other machines no adjustment is needed, but the deflection should be tested as described. The electrocardiogram can then be recorded. On most machines the leads are selected by a rotating switch. This may simply turn from one position to another. Other machines are switched by pulling the switch up to make contact, then pressing it down, turning to the next position and pulling it up once more. In machines of this type, allow at least 3 seconds in the down position before turning to the next place and lifting once more. The electronic system may become unstable if this pause is not made. On other machines, the leads are indicated by a row of push buttons. Here the recording is made by depressing one knob after another along the row. This machine makes its own pause.

The leads are best recorded in the order on the machine, as this simplifies labelling the recording afterwards. The connections the switch makes are:

     I   Right arm to left arm
    II   Right arm to left leg
   III   Left arm to left leg
 AVR   Right arm to left arm and left leg
 AVL   Left arm to right arm and left leg
 AVF   Left leg to right arm and left arm
    V   Chest lead to all three limb leads.

The chest leads are:

V1 Fourth intercostal space at right sternal border
V2 Fourth intercostal space at left sternal border
V3 Half way between V2 and V4
V4 Mid clavicular line in the fifth space
V5 Anterior axillary line, same level V4
V6 Mid axillary line, same level as V4
V   Posterior axillary line, same level as V4.

The sucker for the chest leads should be applied to skin lightly smeared with electrode jelly. This should be put on carefully in spots corresponding to the places described above. When a chest is too hairy for the sucker, hold it in place by the rubber part of the sucker.

In some patients the deflections are too big to go on the paper. When this happens the sensitivity of the machine should be reduced by 1 millivolt to 0·5 cm which is half the normal sensitivity. This is noted on the recording by writing the lead followed by × 2, for example V4 × 2.

Remember that any muscle will produce a voltage change when it contracts. If the patient is not relaxed, the recording will show fine oscillations due to the contractions of the limb and chest muscles.

Finally *ALWAYS* switch the machine off after use. Battery operated machines quickly exhaust the batteries if left switched on.

MONITORING EQUIPMENT

Anyone working in an intensive care unit has to be more or less familiar with the monitoring equipment in use. The essentials of the various instruments are simple enough and adjusting them is far simpler than adjusting the average domestic television receiver. We shall consider here some of the controls likely to be found on any machine, without reference to any particular instrument.

We may begin with a typical ECG monitor with built in rate-meter and alarm system (Fig.34). This consists of the following components all in a single case:

1. An oscilloscope and its controls

2. An ECG amplifier and controls

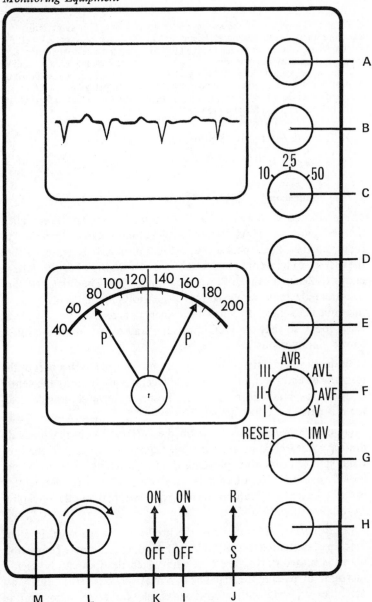

Fig.34. A typical monitoring oscilloscope. The upper display is an oscilloscope showing the electrocardiogram. The lower dial is a ratemeter, in this case a pointer rotating from a spindle. Two pointers on this dial (lettered P & P) can be adjusted to set the limits for triggering the alarm. A = brightness. B = focus.

[*continued overleaf*]

C-Y shift. D = speed of the sweep of the ECG trace. E = gain control for adjusting the voltage response of the ECG. F = lead selector. G = 1 mv standardizing voltage. H = gain control for adjusting the sensitivity of the rate-meter. I = polarity selector for R or S wave to trigger ratemeter. J = audible tick on or off switch. K = alarm signal on or off switch. L = standardizing control for the ratemeter. M = standard 120 beats per minute output for standardizing ratemeter. The mains lead, patient cable and on and off switch are at the rear of the machine and are not shown.

3. The ratemeter and its controls

4. The alarm system and its controls.

1. The oscilloscope

The oscilloscope consists of a phosphorescent screen, often called the phosphor, on which a spot of light moves across from left to right and then flicks back to repeat its journey. It is arranged that the voltage to be recorded deflects the spot upwards when the voltage is positive and downwards when it is negative. The image or spot does not fade immediately, so the screen shows the image as a fading line across its face. In some instruments there may be several of these spots, so that the ECG, pressures and other things can all be shown simultaneously.

In the simplest instruments there are no controls to this part of the instrument and the spot automatically centres itself along the centre of the phosphor. Most machines, however, have several controls for this part of the instrument. The following are common:

(1) *On/off switch*. This turns on the current. Many machines do not have one, while in some it is placed at the rear end of the box. If no spot appears after plugging in and switching on at the main, look fore and aft for a switch labelled 'on' and try that. Remember it may take half a minute to warm up and sweep across the phosphor to stabilize its position.

(2) *Brightness*. This controls the brightness of the spot. In some machines, particularly in a brightly lit ward, the spot may be invisible if this is turned down. The ease with which the spot can be seen is increased by placing the machine in a relatively dark situation. Most machines are sold with a cowl which slots over the phosphor to shade it. This should be kept in place to increase the visibility of the spot on the screen.

(3) *Focus*. This clarifies the spot. It should be adjusted so that the spot is seen as a dot of light with no halo round it.

(4) *Speed.* This controls the rate with which the spot sweeps across the screen. On some models the speed is continuously variable by a knob which turns from fast to slow. On others the switch has positions giving stated sweep speed, usually 10, 25 and 50 mm per second. These correspond to the accepted standard speeds for recording the ECG on paper.

(5) *Y Axis.* This moves the spot up and down. It is usually possible to move the spot off the screen altogether with this control when fitted. Wrong adjustment of this control is therefore a possible reason for no spot appearing after switching on and warming up. The knob should be turned one way and then the other to see if the spot is off the screen. With multi-channel machines, as those with several spots may be called, it is possible to lose a channel because two are exactly superimposed. Gently turning the control for Y axis for each channel in succession will show if this has happened.

(6) *X Axis.* It is unusual to find this control. It controls the centring of the beam on the phosphor from left to right, instead of up and down. When it is not correctly adjusted, the trace is seen on only part of the screen, the remainder remaining blank. It should be adjusted to bring the sweep back on to the screen. If a machine develops this fault and does not have an obvious control, it is best to get an expert to adjust it. There may be an appropriate control hidden under a panel somewhere, but knobs under panels are best left to those who understand them (or they would not have been put under a panel).

2. The electrocardiograph

The electrocardiograph is similar to that in the machines used for ordinary tracings, except that it records on the oscilloscope. There is the usual patient cable with a minimum of three leads. With the three lead type, all three must be attached to the patient. People have various preferences about where to attach them—to the arms, the chest wall or up and down the sternum. It does not matter as long as a good tracing free of interference is obtained. With arm plates a liberal coating of electrode jelly between the plate and the arm is essential, as the arm movement tends to allow the jelly to dry out. This will produce interference on the tracing and, eventually, no record.

Electrodes. The electrodes for attaching to the chest may be made of a metal disc, steel gauze or plate of points like a nutmeg grater.

Some have a sticky surface like a plaster which is protected by a paper coating. This is peeled off and the electrode stuck to the skin. In another type, the electrode is permanently attached to the cable and is stuck on with plaster. With all types, see that the metal surface of the electrode is clean and bright before sticking it. Some metal skin electrodes cause sensitivity reactions in the skin if they are attached for some hours or days. This should be watched for. If the type in use is known to do this, it is safest to make a practice of always placing a little pledget of lint, moistened with electrode jelly, between the metal and the skin. If the skin is covered with much hair as on some chests, the hair should be shaved off. When the lead on the machine is of the standard type with five cables, it is enough to attach the right arm, left arm and right leg leads to the connector plates, which may be placed on the appropriate limbs or on the chest. Such a machine will have a selector switch and position I will give the ECG. In some units it is the practice to attach all the limb leads correctly. This permits the standard leads of the ECG to be recorded at any time, without the need for reconnecting the patient.

Selector switch. This is fitted to any machine using a standard cable. It permits the appropriate lead to be displayed if the patient is correctly wired up. It is not fitted to a three lead machine.

Calibration. This allows the voltage recorded to be standardized. When the spring loaded switch is turned to the position marked calibrate, cal or 1 mv a 1 millivolt pulse is passed into the recorder. It is usually possible to do this with the selector at O. It has little purpose when the machine is being used simply for monitoring, but is essential if a standard ECG is being recorded from the electro-cardiograph, as can be done on some machines (see below).

Sensitivity. This controls the response of the electrocardiograph to voltage change. In monitoring, it is used to adjust the tracing to a convenient size so that it can be easily seen and will trigger the ratemeter. In recording the ECG on paper, it is used to standardize the deflection of the recorder to 1 cm per 1 millivolt deflection.

3. The ratemeter

This device counts the rate of the heart by an electrical response to the deflection of the electrocardiogram. The meter is usually either a needle rotating on a spindle (Fig.30), or a needle moving on a horizontal numbered strip. In either case there is usually an adjustable pointer on either side of the indicator, which sets limits for heart rate at which the alarm goes off. The controls are easily understood if the mechanism is explained.

The usual ECG has a main deflection which is much bigger than all the others. This may be positive (an R wave) or negative (an S wave). The ratemeter has an adjustable sensitivity which should allow it to be triggered by this major deflection, but not by the smaller ones such as the P and T waves. To get it to work, then, an ECG on the oscilloscope is needed, which does have one deflection two or three times bigger than all the others. If the ECG displayed does not have this characteristic, then the position of the electrodes on the chest or the lead selected should be changed until a satisfactory trace is obtained.

Polarity. Having got a satisfactory ECG the next thing is to get the machine to answer to it. Most instruments have a switch labelled R or S wave. If the main deflection on the oscilloscope is upwards, turn the switch to R wave, if downwards to S wave. This *should* mean that the machine will respond to the deflection selected, but experience will show that this expectation is not always realized. For years we had a machine on our unit which always responded the opposite way, possibly because it was wired the wrong way round, and other machines do not seem to care: they respond equally well whichever way the switch is turned.

Sensitivity. This switch determines the size of the voltage deflection to which the ratemeter will respond. Start with it set to its least sensitive and turn up the sensitivity until the ratemeter begins to record. This is most easily done by switching on the monitor to 'audible' (see below) so that the pulses can be heard. When it does so you should see the ratemeter needle begin to move up from its resting position. Wait until it is stable and then check its reading against the heart rate measured by a second hand of a watch, counting the pulses seen on the oscilloscope. They should correspond to within ten beats per minute. If the ratemeter is wrong, for example recording 240 beats per minute instead of 120, then it is picking up an extra pulse. This could be the P wave or the T wave. If adjusting the sensitivity of the ratemeter does not stop the error, it may be possible to get it right by turning up the sensitivity of the ECG and turning down the sensitivity of the meter. Alternatively a different position for the ECG plates may be needed. If, however, the oscilloscope shows a dominant R or S wave, all should be well. Most machines have an arrangement for testing the ratemeter. This is usually a button labelled 'test' with a number (usually 120) beside it. When the button is pressed, 120 pulses a minute are fed into the ratemeter. There is an adjusting knob for correcting the meter. With the machine on but the ECG off, press the knob and wait until the meter stabilizes. If it is not at 120 adjust the meter to read 120, waiting between each adjustment for the meter to stabilize. This part of the instrument is very stable and rarely needs adjustment.

4. The alarm system

At its simplest this consists of an audible bleep in time with the heart beat and a continuous wail if the rate goes outside the limits set by the system on the dial of the ratemeter. There is usually a switch labelled 'silent/audible' which turns on the bleeper and a control knob for the loudness of the signal. A further switch turns the alarm off and on. The snags of having too much of a good thing where bleepers are concerned, have been mentioned earlier. At its most complicated there is a system of coloured lights, all labelled, to tell the nurse if the heart is going too fast, too slow or not going at all. The machine is reminiscent of a pin table but, unfortunately, unlike a pin table does not have an illuminated panel labelled tilt. In other words, its complicated mechanism does not distinguish between the patient going off, or the machine's recording system going off. In all this work the look of the patient comes before the information conveyed by any gadget.

In any system of this kind the efficiency of the warning system depends upon the initial signal sent into it from the ECG. Where a patient is restless or the electrocardiogram of low voltage, the system may fail, either because too many false impulses are entering it or because the ECG does not have a big enough voltage to trigger the ratemeter. In any case no sophistication of the instrument replaces the human eye watching the patient and his electrocardiogram.

The foregoing describes the usual monitoring apparatus. Many elaborations exist. A common one is a direct writing electrocardiograph coupled to the monitoring oscilloscope. This permits the recording of an immediate permanent trace. In some instruments the ECG will print a short recording automatically at selected intervals, while some will start to record automatically if the alarm is triggered. An even more sophisticated arrangement includes a continuous tape recording of the ECG and other data. With this it is possible to play over the events recorded before any alarm was triggered. Some arrangement of this sort is used in many research programmes today for recording the effect of new treatments.

DEFIBRILLATORS

The use of defibrillators has been described earlier. Some details about their use are added here, to enable the nurse to appreciate the differences in procedure which she will see in the management of patients.

Ventricular fibrillation is an emergency in which the ventricles are not contracting and so there is no cardiac output. External cardiac massage will keep the circulation going, but usually the fibrillation persists. A defibrillating shock is most likely to restore the ventricular beat, and, as the ventricles are not contracting the shock may be applied at any time—there is no cardiac cycle. A charge of 100 to 400 joules may be given.

Ventricular tachycardia will also respond to a defibrillation shock, and again the timing in relation to the cardiac cycle does not matter. The voltage needed may be quite small—30 to 100 joules.

Atrial fibrillation requires a more complicated arrangement since the ventricles in this condition are beating normally. If an electric shock is delivered when the ventricular muscle is capable of contraction, it may be provoked to fibrillate. To avoid this, the shock is delivered when the ventricles are in their refractory state and not responsive to stimuli (see page 33). This is shortly after the R wave of the ECG. It will be recalled that the ratemeter is triggered by the R (or S) wave. In the same way, the defibrillator can also be triggered to the ECG and when this is done it will discharge on a signal from the ECG. In setting this up, it is again necessary to make sure that the triggering mechanism is set appropriately for an R wave or an S wave, whichever is the main deflection in the ECG. The condenser is charged up, the defibrillating plates applied to the chest wall of the patient, who is preferably anaesthetized, and the defibrillation button pressed down and kept down. Immediately after the next R (or S) wave on the ECG the machine will fire.

A final word about electrical apparatus, particularly defibrillators. Accidental discharge of electrical currents through medical or nursing staff, can cause cardiac standstill or ventricular fibrillation. Handle all apparatus with caution and if an accident does occur remember the cause, if a defibrillator, may be the cure. There are many people working today who have had an accidental shock from a defibrillator or electric cautery in theatre which has caused ventricular fibrillation. The application of a second shock from a defibrillator has restored normal cardiac action—and the person concerned has been on duty next day.

SALINE MANOMETER

This consists of a simple plastic tube connected to the infusion line by a 3-way tap. To use it to record atrial pressure, first turn the tap to position A. The manometer tube will fill to the height of the reservoir. Now turn to position B. The saline in the mano-meter will fall to the level of the atrial pressure, and should show slight rises and falls in time with respiration. If a respiratory oscillation is not seen, the end of the tube is likely to be blocked. either by clot or because it is pressed against the lining of the heart, After recording the pressure, turn the tap to position C to continue the infusion. This sequence should always be used. The simpler method of turning the tap from C to B without first filling the manometer as at A, will result in the manometer filling with blood

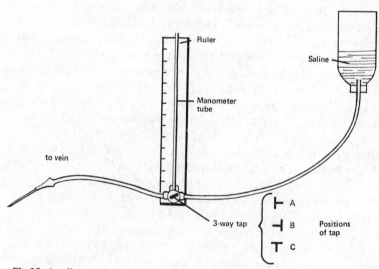

Fig.35. A saline manometer, E. reservoir, F plastic tubing, G tap, H manometer tube of clear plastic tubing, I ruler, J intravenous fine bore tubing, A, B & C different tap positions.

if the atrial pressure is high. This may result in the saline infusion tube being rendered useless by blood clot. Always hold the manometer tube vertical when noting pressure (see page 107).

Index